Feeling Unreal

Feeling Unreal

Depersonalization and the Loss of the Self

Second Edition

DAPHNE SIMEON, MD AND JEFFREY ABUGEL

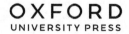

OXFORD
UNIVERSITY PRESS

OXFORD
UNIVERSITY PRESS

Oxford University Press is a department of the University of Oxford. It furthers
the University's objective of excellence in research, scholarship, and education
by publishing worldwide. Oxford is a registered trade mark of Oxford University
Press in the UK and certain other countries.

Published in the United States of America by Oxford University Press
198 Madison Avenue, New York, NY 10016, United States of America.

Library of Congress Cataloging-in-Publication Data
Names: Simeon, Daphne, 1958– author. | Abugel, Jeffrey, author.
Title: Feeling unreal : depersonalization and the loss of the self /
Daphne Simeon, MD and Jeffrey Abugel.
Description: Second edition. | New York, NY : Oxford University Press, [2023] |
Includes bibliographical references and index.
Identifiers: LCCN 2022053526 (print) | LCCN 2022053527 (ebook) |
ISBN 9780197622445 (paperback) | ISBN 9780197622469 (epub) |
ISBN 9780197622476
Subjects: LCSH: Depersonalization. | Identity (Psychology)
Classification: LCC RC553.D4 S56 2023 (print) | LCC RC553.D4 (ebook) |
DDC 155.2—dc23/eng/20221202
LC record available at https://lccn.loc.gov/2022053526
LC ebook record available at https://lccn.loc.gov/2022053527

DOI: 10.1093/oso/9780197622445.001.0001

1 3 5 7 9 8 6 4 2

Printed by Sheridan Books, Inc., United States of America

To my children.
—Daphne Simeon

To family and friends who have supported me through the years.
—Jeffrey Abugel

Contents

Preface

When *Feeling Unreal: Depersonalization and the Loss of the Self* appeared in 2006, it was praised as a seminal work—the first book providing a comprehensive overview of the baffling condition then known as depersonalization disorder. The world has changed dramatically since. To some degree, what is now known as depersonalization/derealization disorder (DDD) is emerging from the shadows of obscurity, through continuing and expanding scientific inquiry as well as an explosion of social media. Major articles about DDD have appeared in print in the *Washington Post*, *Atlantic Monthly*, *Elle*, and *The Guardian*. The feature film *Numb*, starring Matthew Perry, brought the disorder into mainstream culture. In some quarters, the social isolation resulting from the COVID-19 lockdown brought depersonalization to the forefront of concern and discussion. And yet DDD's obscurity is slow to fade, and the condition remains relatively unknown or unacknowledged by many in the medical and other mental health communities.

Whether documented yesterday or a century ago, the core symptoms of DDD remain unchanged. Many people have felt "unreal" at some point in life, albeit fleetingly. For people with DDD, the world within, or the world around, is experienced as strange and unreal for prolonged periods of time. They feel detached from the sense of self they once took for granted and they struggle, sometimes for years, in search of answers, which can be difficult to come by. Imagine thinking without feeling, devoid of emotional connection to past or present. Imagine a heightened awareness of the thoughts parading through your head, or always watching yourself a step removed, interrupted periodically by a single emotion—the real fear of losing your mind. Living this way, vacuous, numb, and lost, wreaks havoc on individuals' inner lives. Outwardly they may appear rather normal, even well adjusted. But they know something is wrong, though they may not know what it is, so their lives often become façades of normalcy, masks to cover the unreality within.

The second edition of *Feeling Unreal* aims to present and discuss all that we now know about DDD, nearly two decades after the first edition. Our intention is to present a comprehensive and unbiased distillation of the broadening range of scientific material that has addressed depersonalization/

derealization to date, as well as to examine the many philosophical, literary, religious, and spiritual reflections on depersonalized-like states of mind. *Feeling Unreal* is the culmination of decades of work seeking answers to questions that have remained elusive or unsynthesized for too long. As such, we hope that the book will be a valuable resource for sufferers and their loved ones, clinicians, students of depersonalization across disciplines, and all others intrigued by the state of mind that uniquely straddles psychopathology and being.

1

Strangers to Ourselves

We do not see things as they are, we see them as we are.

—Anaïs Nin

The idea that reality is subjective, constructed from our own perceptions, is an ancient concept. "We are what we think. All that we are arises with our thoughts. With our thoughts, we make the world," said the Buddha. In the same vein, Anaïs Nin's observation above originated in the Hebrew Talmud.

But what if our perceptions of our own thoughts, or the world around us, change in an inexplicable way? What if the world suddenly seems strange, and foreign? This is the story of a baffling but very real condition of the mind that plagues millions of people worldwide. It isn't depression, or anxiety, though it can sometimes appear as a symptom of these better-known conditions. Often, it emerges with cruel ferocity as a chronic disorder completely unto itself. Its destructive impact on an individual's sense of self is implied in its very name—depersonalization.

Depersonalization/derealization disorder (DDD) is a serious disruption in a person's experience of the self that alters their entire world. Take the case of Ron, a 39-year-old magazine editor living in a coastal city. To his peers, Ron's life is practically heaven on earth. He's bright, funny, and successful at his job. With an apartment near the beach and plenty of friends, he is living a life that is envied by many. But Ron has a problem. And each day when he returns to his upscale neighborhood in time to see the sun setting, he wonders how long he can maintain what he has. He wonders if tonight will be the night he finally slips into the isolated hell of insanity.

Ron's problem is a mental one, and he knows it. Trapped within the confines of his mind, he is too aware of every thought passing through it, as if he were outside, looking in. At night he often lies awake ruminating endlessly about what's wrong with him, about death, and about the meaning of existence itself. At times his arms and legs feel like they don't belong with his

Feeling Unreal. Second Edition. Daphne Simeon and Jeffrey Abugel, Oxford University Press. © Oxford University Press 2023. DOI: 10.1093/oso/9780197622445.003.0001

body. But most of the time, his mind feels like it is operating apart from the body that contains it.

While he can interact with others who have no idea that anything is wrong, Ron lives without spontaneity, going through the motions, doing what he thinks people expect him to, glad that he is able to at least *appear* normal throughout the day and maintain a job. He studied drama briefly while in college and remained enamored of Shakespeare and literature, but an emerging self-consciousness eventually robbed him of his ability to act. Now he feels as if *all* of his life is an act—just an attempt to maintain the status quo.

Recalling literature he once loved, he sometimes pictures himself as Camus's Meursault, in *The Stranger*, an emotionless character who plods through life in a meaningless universe with apathy and indifference. He's tired of living this way but terrified of death. So he's settled into a predictable routine whereby work serves as a necessary diversion, and happiness is a dearly departed illusion. Dead people can't be happy, he thinks. To be happy, one has to feel, and Ron has not felt anything but fear, confusion, and despair for a long time.

In his autobiographical account of his battle with debilitating depression, *Darkness Visible*, William Styron writes: "Depression is a disorder of mood, so mysteriously painful and elusive in the way it becomes known to the self— to the mediating intellect—as to verge close to being beyond description."[1] The writer's skills are tested when writing about what Styron calls "a shipwreck of the mind." The wreckage caused by depersonalization is equally indescribable to anyone who has not experienced it. Phrases like "things feel unreal to me," "I feel detached from myself," and "my voice sounds different to me" are enigmatic to normal people yet often quite understandable to depersonalized individuals.

Most of us can imagine our darkest fear, such as being buried alive, or locked in a room full of rats or spiders. Most of us can remember moments of intolerable grief or unbridled terror, whether they occurred in waking life or in nightmares. We can remember being unable to "shake" some awful sensation in the conscious hours after a particularly bad dream, or feeling "unreal" in the face of a sudden tragedy or loss. For the most part, depersonalized people are actually living every day with the fear and unreality of a dream state come true. Inner and outer worlds seem strange and foreign, resulting in an altered sense of selfhood that dominates their mental lives.

Our sense of familiarity with ourselves, our sense of past, present, or future, who we are, and how we fit into the world around us enables us to live from day to day in relative stability, with purpose, sanity, and reason. But people with chronic depersonalization are never quite sure who they are, in a sense. As such, they can find themselves in a life of going through the motions robotically, often attempting to appear "normal," wondering if others can see through their façade to the inexplicable disconnection that pervades their existence.

Tom, a 44-year-old sales executive, feels that he gets through his job using about 10% of his brain capacity:

> I'll sit in an important meeting and be asked crucial questions, and somehow I come up with the answers. But I'm not really there. It's as if nothing is real, myself or the meeting I am in. I look out the window 40 stories up and wonder where the sky ends. Or I see myself sitting in this meeting, discussing bottom lines and sales promotions as if they actually had meaning to me. It's more than daydreaming. It's like I'm too aware of certain larger aspects of reality. In the face of the infinite sky above me, or infinite time before and after my short existence, how could such things as my job have any meaning at all? Doesn't anyone else ever wonder about this stuff?

Tom's sense of detachment from everything that is immediate and vivid in the day-to-day world, and his over-preoccupation with the nature of existence, is something often experienced by depersonalized people. Says Cheryl, a 33-year-old fabric designer:

> I sometimes feel like I'm from Mars.... Being human seems strange, bodily functions seem bizarre . . . My thoughts seem separate from my body. At times, the most common, familiar objects can seem foreign, as if I am looking at them for the first time. An American flag, for instance. It's instantly recognizable, and immediately means something to everyone. But if I look at it for more than a moment, I just see colors and shapes on a piece of cloth. It's as if I've forgotten ever seeing the flag before, even though I'm still aware of what my "normal" reaction should be.

This sense of strangeness about familiar objects outside of one's self is known specifically as *derealization*, the flip side of the depersonalization experience. "What's so troubling to me is that if I were seeing these things for the first time, like a child, there should be some sense of wonderment, but there isn't," Cheryl adds. "I know that there's something wrong with me, and all it does is fill me with fear, especially the fear of being taken away screaming in a straitjacket."

Louise is a 29-year-old grade school teacher whose experiences of depersonalization permeate all the ways in which she relates to her body and her movements, as well as her whole visual experience of the world. Her depersonalization started when she was around 10, at which time she felt that whenever she lifted up her legs or arms, her body felt weightless, and she began to float. She says: "For me, it can be a very visual experience. It's like I'm wearing glasses that I can't see through, like there is a zipper to unzip." She no longer feels much; she describes herself as numb, and it's rare for her to cry even when she feels like it. Her body does not feel like a part of her: "I sometimes smack my hand or pinch my leg just to feel something, and to know it's there." Louise often feels like one part of her is "acting." At the same time, "there is another part 'inside' that is not connecting with the *me* that is talking to you," she says. When the depersonalization is at its most intense, she feels like she just does not exist. These experiences leave her confused about who she really is, and quite often she feels like an "actress" or simply "a fake."

Phil, 42, owns a successful business and is the father of two. He first experienced depersonalization when he was 17, and in the beginning the episodes would come and go. For the past 15 years or so, however, his depersonalization has been constant, at times more intense than at others. Like Louise, he eloquently describes the many facets of his self-experience that have become chronically distorted by depersonalization. He has thought about his condition a great deal and has researched it on his own, as fervently as any doctor he has met to date. When he tries to explain his experiences to a professional, or to someone close to him, he does so in terms of the distinct domains of his selfhood that are affected:

Emotions: "I want to feel things like everyone else again, but I'm deadened and numb. I can laugh or cry but it's intellectual; my muscles move but I feel nothing."

Body: "I feel like I'm not here, I'm floating around. A separate part of me is aware of all my movements; it's like I've left my body. Even when I'm talking I don't feel like it is my words."

Mind: "My mind and my body are somehow not connected; it's like my body is doing one thing and my mind is saying another. Like my mind is somewhere off to the back, not inside my body."

Vision: "It's like glass over my eyes, a visual fog totally flat and two-dimensional."

Agency: "I feel I'm not really here, I'm not in control of my actions. I'm just going through the motions, like a robot."

People like Phil may suffer from chronic DDD for many years, visiting a variety of doctors, psychiatrists, and therapists. Typically, health professionals are not only unable to offer much relief, but they rarely even offer a reassuring label for the condition. Patients are commonly told that they suffer from some kind of anxiety or depression and that what they feel is secondary to their main problem.

The frightening absence of feeling often encountered in DDD also can create a somewhat paradoxical state of mind. On one hand, selfhood, and with it the individual's relation to the outer world, seems to deteriorate, leaving the sensation of "no-self." Conversely, a heightened awareness of inner experiences, like the thoughts running through one's head, or visceral sensations that cannot be ignored, can result in a hyper-monitoring of the self, a self that no longer feels familiar, grounded, or unquestioned. Strongly held desires and beliefs, vivid memories, strong emotions that were naturally sparked by the senses now all seem like illusions, far away, without real meaning, somehow false. Familiar mental images are reduced to movie-screen images devoid of the smells, sounds, and punch that once made them click. Ideas and memories that once had emotional meaning are now experienced with alien-like awareness and little feeling, while the sufferer remains intellectually aware that this altered perspective is anything but normal. This lack of "embeddedness" that accompanies a normal sense of self can leave one feeling lost, vulnerable, and fearful.

"When I try to explain this, it sounds like a complete contradiction," says Joanne, a 35-year-old mother of three. "Minutes can seem like hours to me when every thought, no matter how insignificant, is weighed and overly present. It's like my thoughts are on a big movie screen in huge type, or shouted at me in a loud unpleasant voice. Yet at the same time, my lifetime, and all the lifetimes before and after mine, seem to last just seconds in the scheme of things. I try to recapture the feeling I had when I was young, that life was rich with promise. I looked forward to building memories to cherish in my old age. But now it all seems so short and empty, as if all the experiences I did enjoy to this point have been erased and I'm just existing in this very second . . . there is no past, no future. Instead of being rooted in this world, enjoying my children and my life, all I can think of is how transient it all is."

"I'd really rather have cancer than this," Joanne concludes. And she's not alone in this sentiment: others who are chronically depersonalized have made the exact same statement. "With a disease that people know, you get some degree of empathy. But if you try to explain this, people either think you're crazy or completely self-absorbed and neurotic. So you keep your mouth shut and suffer silently." Indeed, depersonalized individuals often say they would give anything to live their lives again with less scrutiny of existence and more spontaneity. While Socrates may have concluded that "the unexamined life is not worth living," the *overly* examined life, as experienced by the people we've met so far, is often too painful to endure.

Hardly a New Disorder

Depersonalization, as a human experience, is nothing new. It has traditionally been viewed as the mind's natural way of coping with overwhelming shock or stress, or intolerably inhumane living conditions. In such instances, the mind detaches itself from the surroundings for the purpose of sheer survival. But strangely, depersonalization can also appear spontaneously, without any apparent trigger. Possible causes of onset have only been researched in depth in the past couple of decades, though theories have proliferated for over a century (we'll cover these causes in more detail later). Some people can recall exactly how and when the problem began and whether or not it was tied to a specific event. For others, the condition may have begun so early in life that it is simply all they have ever known. In such cases, depersonalization becomes a safe void where nothing affects them, but at high price: when they'd like to feel, they can't. They become what some have come to call "the living dead."

The word *depersonalization* itself, in a diagnostic sense, refers to both symptoms and to the full-blown psychiatric disorder of DDD. Ludovic Dugas, a psychologist and philosopher who often wrote on the topics of memory and déjà vu, is most often credited with first using the term in its present context, in the late 1890s.[2] However, Dugas had first seen the word in a popular literary work of the era, *The Journal Intime*, by Henri Frédéric Amiel (1821–1881). This journal, the voluminous diary of an introspective and obscure professor, was published posthumously. One particular entry helped to define the nature of depersonalization for all time: "And now I find myself regarding existence as though beyond the tomb, from another world. All is strange to me; I am, as it were, outside my own body and individuality; I am depersonalized, detached, cut adrift. Is this madness?"[3]

Other more renowned individuals later recognized depersonalization/derealization (dpdr) as very concrete human experiences. Sigmund Freud experienced a vivid encounter with derealization while visiting the Acropolis during a trip to Athens in 1904.[4] We'll take a closer look at Freud's experience, as well as dpdr's presence in psychology, history, and philosophy, in subsequent chapters.

In years that followed, renowned psychologists either touched on the subject of dpdr in books or issued lengthy papers on it in nearly every major language. In the 1930s, a medical textbook entitled *Modern Clinical Psychiatry* first included depersonalization within the context of schizophrenia. Revised years later in the 1960s, it provided a particularly insightful description:

> Depersonalization, a pervasive and distressing feeling of estrangement, known sometimes as the depersonalization syndrome, may be defined as an affective disorder in which feelings of unreality and a loss of conviction of one's own identity and of a sense of identification with and control over one's own body are the principal symptoms. The unreality symptoms are of two kinds: a feeling of changed personality and a feeling that the outside world is unreal. The patient feels that he is no longer himself, but he does not feel that he has become someone else. The condition is, therefore, not one of so-called transformation of personality. Experience loses emotional meaning and may be colored by a frightening sense of strangeness and unreality. The onset may be acute, following a severe emotional shock, or it may be a gradual onset following prolonged physical or emotional stress. It is more frequent in personalities of an intelligent, sensitive, affectionate, introverted, and imaginative type. The patient may say his feelings are "frozen," that his thoughts are strange; his thoughts and acts seem to be carried on mechanically as if he were a machine or automaton. People and objects appear unreal, far away, and lacking in normal color and vividness. The patient may say he feels as if he were going about in a trance or dream. He appears perplexed and bewildered because of the strangeness of unreality feelings. He has difficulty in concentrating and may complain that his brain is "dead" or has "stopped working."[5]

To be accurate in terms of what's known today, the description should have ended there. But, in line with older theories about depersonalization, the textbook postulated that depersonalization was not a specific condition outside of other neurotic and psychotic states and that it occurred more commonly in women and in puberty, and recommended electroshock therapy as the effective form of treatment. Times and attitudes have changed. It is now thought that the condition occurs about equally across genders, at many stages of life. Chronic dpdr is now recognized as a unique disorder of its own standing, depersonalization/derealization disorder (DDD), rather than a condition secondary to other ailments.

Unlike the early days of studying the mind, today's field of psychiatry has developed a reference book, the *Diagnostic and Statistical Manual of Psychiatric Disorders (DSM)*, revised periodically to stay current. These revisions list the latest criteria for making an accurate diagnosis of virtually any known mental illness based on more recently gathered evidence. Early versions of the *DSM* from the 1950s and 1960s mentioned depersonalization as a dissociative reaction or syndrome, classified in the category of neurotic disorders. From 1980 on, chronic depersonalization was placed within the new category of dissociative disorders, yet the *DSM* offered few specifics about the condition. But today that's changed. According to the latest edition, *DSM-5-TR*,[6] DDD is described as follows.

An individual suffering from depersonalization may experience:

- Detachment from one's whole self or from aspects of the self.
- Detachment from feelings.
- Detachment from thoughts.
- Detachment from the whole body or body parts.
- Detachment from sensations.
- Diminished sense of agency.
- A split self, one part observing and one participating.

Sufferers of derealization may experience:

- Detachment from the world (people, objects, or all surroundings).
- Feeling as if one is in a fog, dream, or bubble.
- The sensation of a veil or glass between the self and the world around.
- Surroundings that seem artificial, colorless, or lifeless.

- Visual distortions (blurriness, changes in visual field, dimensionality, or size of objects).
- Auditory distortions (voices or sounds are muted or heightened).

Patients may experience symptoms of one or both elements for a diagnosis of DDD to be made. And symptoms may be episodic or recurring (see Chapters 3 and 4 for more about symptoms and diagnosis). *Unreality* and *detachment* are the essence of dpdr, despite the multitude of symptoms that have been recorded over time. People may have difficulty describing their symptoms and may fear that their experiences in fact signify that they are losing their mind, going "crazy."

At some point in their lives, many adults will experience a brief episode of dpdr, usually precipitated by severe stress or trauma. Depersonalization has been found to occur transiently in one-third to one-half of student populations.[7] Transient depersonalization, lasting seconds, minutes, or even hours, can readily occur in otherwise "healthy" individuals under extreme conditions of sleep deprivation, sensory deprivation, travel to unknown places, or acute intoxication with marijuana or hallucinogens. It also occurs in about one-third of people who have been exposed to life-threatening danger, and about 10% of patients hospitalized for various mental disorders.[8] Depersonalization has been found to occur, at least fleetingly, in 50% to 70% of the general population.[9] Most often, initial depersonalization goes away as mysteriously as it came, but sometimes it becomes more chronic, with an enigmatic life of its own. Research shows that approximately 2% of the general population suffers from chronic depersonalization that rises to the level of a psychiatric disorder.[9]

Sudden depersonalization is likely to make a person think they're going insane. When it occurs after they've taken an illicit drug, they often think they've suffered brain damage. No longer grounded by familiar sensations or surroundings, they feel as if they're losing their grip on reality. But unlike people with psychotic conditions like schizophrenia, they are not going insane at all. They are, if anything, suddenly *overly aware* of reality and existence and of the ways in which their own experience is a distortion of the "normal" sense of a real self.

Depersonalization, in fact, resembles a sort of altered "consciousness," akin to the "awakening" that in some cultures is thought to be a level of spiritual growth. This is touched upon in the *DSM-5-TR*, which distinguishes the condition from mental states that are actively sought out, often through meditation. But for most "Westerners," this abnormal sense of having no self is a state they'd prefer to leave behind (in Chapter 9, we'll take a closer look at philosophical and spiritual interpretations of this state of mind).

The Madness of the New Millennium?

Exploration of the nature of dpdr, as a transient symptom or as a full-blown chronic disorder, is now taking on a new importance for several reasons. First, the use of illicit drugs, from the 1960s until now, has fostered an explosion of depersonalization cases in the last 50 years. Marijuana, legal or not, and other drugs such as hallucinogens and Ecstasy are well known to sometimes trigger chronic depersonalization. Second, there is evidence that more people are experiencing depersonalization, or making it known, than ever before, whatever the initial precipitant. Many of these people have suffered in silence, perplexity, isolation, and shame for years. Then, the advent of the internet prompted the founding of several depersonalization support group websites. Consequently, thousands of people with strikingly similar experiences and symptoms began congregating in the late 1990s with a hunger for information and comfort through this new venue. One of the earliest websites, depersonalization.info, has received more than 200,000 hits since its creation in 2002. The posting below is typical of the personal stories contributed by people who visit briefly, then return to their solitary worlds:

> I look at my mind from within and feel both trapped and puzzled about the strangeness of my existence. My thoughts swirl round and round constantly probing the strangeness of selfhood—why do I exist? Why am I me and not someone else? At these times, feelings of sweaty panic develop, as if I am having a phobia about my own thoughts. At other times, I don't feel "grounded." I look at this body and can't understand why I am within it. I hear myself having conversations and wonder where the voice is coming from. I imagine myself seeing life as if it were played like a film in a cinema. But in that case, where am I? Who is watching the film? What is the cinema? The worst part is that this seems as if it's the truth, and the periods of my life in which I did not feel like this were delusions.

This articulate, electronic expression of the strangeness of depersonalization could have come right out of Amiel's journal, written with pen and ink, or from dozens of other philosophical or literary works through the ages. These cries for help did not go unnoticed. In the 1990s, a few medical institutions established research programs singly devoted to the study of DDD. These included the Depersonalization and Dissociation Research Program at the Mount Sinai School of Medicine in New York, and the Depersonalization Research Unit at the Institute of Psychiatry, King's College, London. These programs were devoted to studying depersonalization in depth in all its aspects, and to experimenting with new treatments that might offer relief to those who found DDD an unbearable condition. Many of their findings are examined in later chapters.

Throughout this book we will present numerous personal stories from people suffering from dpdr. Some individuals can trace its onset to a specific trigger such as childhood maltreatment, or traumatic stress, or drug use. Others may not be able to pinpoint when or where their encounter with DDD began with any precision. Some may endure unbearable anxiety, while others feel no anxiety at all. In any case, what they experience falls within the guidelines for a diagnosis of DDD. The detailed case of Alex that follows is one story of many.

The Story of Alex

From his earliest years, Alex felt destined for a life at sea. Growing up in a depressed neighborhood in New York, his greatest pleasures were regular drives to the beach or deep-sea fishing trips with his father or friends. His parents were strict and religious but also loving and fair. They successfully raised him with virtues of honesty and tolerance that would later be admired by many with whom he sailed.

Alex graduated from the U.S. Merchant Marine Academy with honors in the late 1960s and immediately found work as a third officer aboard a large tanker owned by a major oil company. Alex functioned comfortably in a world of order, respect for authority, and a well-founded regard for the inherent power and danger of the oceans of the world.

While the culture he left on land was now obsessed with the Vietnam war, sexual experimentation, drugs, and long hair, there was nothing novel about any of this to men who sailed the ocean regularly. Alex had seen people in

India with hair that had never been cut; he had witnessed bloody skirmishes, even an execution in Africa; and sailors ashore were known for their wanton disregard for conventional morality. Despite many temptations, however, Alex chose to remain morally upright, partly because of his religious beliefs and partly because of the status he needed to maintain in front of the crew.

He had met his wife, Teresa, shortly before graduating, at a Sunday night church service held near the academy. Long love letters between Alex and Teresa accumulated during his earliest voyages, and within a year they were married, despite his mother's protestations. Together they purchased a small house on Long Island, New York.

Between voyages Alex had plenty of time at home and plenty of cash because his expenses on land had been minimal. It was his choice when he sailed again. But some of the major oil and shipping companies, where his friends and classmates worked, were beckoning. He had quickly earned a reputation as an officer with superior navigation and piloting skills, which better assured an uneventful voyage for the monolithic, costly company vessels. He had also been certified for increased responsibility. By his late 20s he was qualified to be a first mate on the largest vessels in the world with only the captain above him.

The first few stays at home with Teresa, after his regular four-month voyages, were like extended honeymoons. But the down payment on the house and subsequent furnishings soon diminished his cash reserves. In time, life on land seemed somewhat unsettling as well. At sea, an officer's authority was like that of a god. On land, people had little respect for authority, were detached from the real power of nature, and were generally ignorant of the realities of life in the rest of the world.

Teresa, who had once promised to continue her education and finish college, also began to change. She no longer exhibited much ambition except for wanting to have children as soon as possible. The couple had talked of parenthood, but they had agreed to wait a few years. But Teresa was impatient; her other friends all had babies with fathers who worked in the city and came home each night. It became clear that this was what she desired as well.

After several voyages to the Far East and South America, Alex began to feel increasingly uneasy during the months spent at home. His ship's cabin had become a compact sanctuary that called for his return. In the new suburban home, Teresa watched too much television and talked on the phone to her parents and friends to an annoying degree. Alex often went to the beach to surf cast, and sometimes prayed for a sign of what to do next. The relationship was strained within the parameters of marriage; it was so different from the days of dating and dreaming of the future. Finally, under pressure from Teresa and her parents, he told her that he would complete one last voyage, then look for maritime-related work on land. An infusion of cash and a break from each other seemed to be what both of them needed.

Alex's last voyage was on Lake Superior, serving as first mate aboard a moderately sized tanker. The money was good, but for Alex, the voyage was uneasy. He didn't know any of the officers or crew and the waters were rough much of the time. He had never worked for this company before and sensed some tendencies to take shortcuts with maintenance and safety. Still, he did his job, remained businesslike, and kept to himself.

On the return voyage, with only days to go, Alex felt inexplicably uneasy again, though some of his distress could be pinned to concern about the future. He was at the moment tired of being on ships, but life on land held little appeal. Perhaps his marriage had been a mistake. His mother had discouraged it; maybe she, as usual, had been right.

Then, in the early morning hours after his four-hour watch, Alex stood outside on the deck to think and perhaps pray. The lake was now placid and glasslike, uncharacteristically still. A fog had rolled in so that the water blended with the horizon to create a single, indeterminate mass. An unsettling stillness overtook Alex as well. His mind was a complete blank, as if awaiting a thought, or a vision. Then, in an instant, he felt something he had never experienced before—an intense sense of panic and fear that seemed to physically begin somewhere in the interior regions of his body and work its way up through his spine into his head. A sharp, blinding fear that he could never have imagined had him looking at the rail before him with a complete and all-encompassing urge to jump over the side.

Stories of madness have always been part of the lore of the sea. Such anecdotes were common in sailing times, when scurvy, poisoning from tin cans, or year-long voyages would trigger serious mental illness in many sailors. Even today, Alex can recall instances of seamen going berserk, having "the fits," or jumping overboard to commit suicide.

His immediate thought on the deck was that this was "his turn." This was what it was like to go insane. The fear was so inextricably intense that his only desire was complete obliteration. It was a fear not of anything that existed before him, nor in the past or future of a life that was unfolding. It was a fear of existence itself. "It was something like waking up to find that you're in a coffin, buried alive," he recalls. "Only the coffin is your body, your very existence."

Physically shaken, Alex raced to his cabin, only to find himself frantically looking around in all directions as if to search for some anchor upon which he could hook his sanity. He sat on his bunk and glanced at the pictures of his wife and parents. He took deep breaths, and after some time the absolute panic began to subside. Was he going insane? Was this what it was like? Had he been poisoned or given LSD by this suspect crew? His mind raced for explanations until, exhausted, he feel asleep.

Alex would never be completely the same again, though he would know some periods of normalcy, or something close to it, in time. He returned home safely and was now glad to be in his own house with Teresa by his side. But his head did not feel right. He felt anxious and fearful of having another attack like the one he'd had on deck. His confidence and self-esteem were gone, and he lay awake all night thinking endlessly about infinity of time and space, the nature of God, and the strangeness of his own existence. All the things he had accomplished, all the places he had been now seemed like dreams, acted out by someone else. He was a fearful, lost, nonperson—the *real* Alex, who had existed beneath the façade of faith, courage, and action for so many years.

Teresa noticed a difference, too. He couldn't make love and had difficulty showing interest in anything she said. Before long he went to see an internist whom he had known for years. A complete physical revealed nothing out of the ordinary. The doctor said it sounded like some kind of depression and anxiety and, after going through his *Physicians' Desk Reference*, prescribed one of the older class of antidepressants.

Over a period of weeks, the medicine did have some effect. At first Alex was sleepy most of the time and took long naps, looking forward to escaping life in dreamless slices of nonexistence. In time, the free-floating anxiety was quelled, and Alex felt he was actually somewhat better. The beginnings of hope began to emerge, but still his thinking seemed somehow separate from the rest of his body. He was able to smile and begin to plan for the future, but he felt like his mind was a radio that was not quite tuned into a station—noise and static and confusion often filled his head with an exhausting over-awareness of every small thing that went on within it.

"In the very beginning, even when the panic had subsided, I never had a mood," Alex recalls. "Everything felt was moment to moment, with every thought overly conscious in my head. I went through numerous variations of this for about a year," he recalls. "I was able to function again, but only in the daily hope that I would wake up one day and be myself again."

Alex's sense of time seemed somehow altered as well. Minutes some-times seemed like hours; yet his whole life now seemed to have raced by him in seconds. In the midst of all this, time continued on its own pace and a decade came and went. On the surface, life looked good. Teresa got the boy and girl she had wanted, and Alex joined up with an old classmate to start a charter fishing boat service on Long Island. The family moved to an established middle-class neighborhood on the South Shore and everyone appeared happy and prosperous. But inside, Alex's private world, hellish at times, continued.

When he felt better from the antidepressants, he stopped taking them with no apparent ill effects. He was no longer the person he once was but tried to somehow be content within the context of what he had become. If things got rough again he could always go back to the medicine and sleep a few days away and make another comeback of sorts.

For more than 10 years, well into the 1980s, Alex kept an encrypted diary documenting what he felt and thought. Over the course of time, there seemed to be some pattern to his condition. If his ailment had specific symptoms that appeared regularly, there might actually be a name for the condition, he rea-soned. With the analytic nature that he had not lost, he determined that he was indeed human and, as such, could only be susceptible to known human ailments. After all, even though he often felt like it, he wasn't from another planet.

To explore this reasoning, and also seek something even more effec-tive than the one antidepressant he had tried, he visited a psychiatrist. Unfortunately, he learned little more than he had from the internist he had seen years earlier. The psychiatrist also suggested long-term psychoanalysis, which Alex viewed with skepticism, if not outright contempt. So he decided to continue on his own. In his diary he broke down his specific symptoms and concluded that they were sometimes predictable, even cyclical. This is how he described his symptoms:

- Free floating anxiety that comes and goes, with a fear of the Panic. This is the direct antithesis of how I once felt, when I was filled with a sense of adventure, confidence, and willingness to go anywhere, do anything.
- Circular, pointless rumination about everything from existence itself to something someone said, to the reasons for my illness.

- Detachment of my inner voice from my body. Almost constantly, the thoughts running through my head are loud and visible and completely detached from my head. They seem up high in my head, somewhere else. The act of thinking seems strange and foreign.
- The Aloneness. An acute awareness of being alone in my thoughts, a prisoner in my own head. A shattering realization that no one, ever, has shared my thoughts with me. I have heard them alone since I was born and will hear them alone until I die.
- Fear of controlling my actions. I drive and wonder what prevents me from intentionally crashing. I play with my children and wonder what keeps me from slaughtering them.
- Over self-consciousness. In crowds, at the mall, at parties, virtually anywhere, I am flustered by noise and crowds and feel that I stick out like an ogre to be mocked in some way. My legs and arms move awkwardly and feel foreign.
- The Voice. The exaggerated self-consciousness initially felt like I was seeing *through* myself all the time, as if someone was watching my every move and making fun. In time, this manifested itself in the form of an actual second voice in my head. For everything I thought on my own, this little voice would make comments, usually derisive ones. This strange presence persisted for about a year and seemed to replace all the other symptoms. Everything was distilled into this second voice, which made my life miserable, despite the fact that I knew that somehow, it was me doing it. When it tried the medication again, it seemed to shrivel up and disappear.

These core symptoms that Alex experienced sometimes appeared concurrently, but most often a single one would manifest itself to the exclusion of all others. When he was panicky, there was no voice. When he felt the aloneness most, anxiety was minimal, except as a direct result of fearing the aloneness. And through it all, he never considered himself depressed. He dealt with that particular annoyance any way he could until either a degree of normalcy or the next symptom took its turn. In time he also learned something quite amazing. In periods of severe stress or heartache, such as when loved ones died or catastrophic events hovered near, he became the "strong one" and dealt far better with it than others around him. In contrast, the smaller daily stresses of life—financial problems, screaming kids, house or car problems, bills, and noise—were difficult to handle, and whenever they were compounded, one or more of his symptoms was sure to emerge.

It's now been decades since that fateful morning on Lake Superior when a first officer's life was changed forever not because of something outside, but rather something deep within. Alex worries little, but feels little. A kind of emotional deadness inside seems to be the end result of a thousand mental blows through the years—and with it, a philosophical interpretation, of sorts.

"That sailor and everything he believed in so strongly no longer exists," Alex says. "And neither do I. I feel like the 'I,' for lack of a better term, is now somehow situated across many moments. My identity is scattered everywhere; as if I am everyone, and everything, and the spaces between things. And there is a sense of loss, because if this feeling is true, I ought to know everything, feel everything, but I don't. It's like the reflection of the sun being split into shards of light on the sea. I have dissolved, into a kind of 'oneness' with all that exists, but it's a fragmented oneness. It isn't yet complete."

Alex's experience mimics those of countless others for whom ongoing stresses may have triggered dpdr, assuming some preexisting predisposition was in place. The symptoms he describes fall into a category that has sometimes been called the "phobic anxiety-depersonalization syndrome," and parallel those described in some of the literature dealing with depersonalization that had appeared in the late 1950s and early 1960s. Unfortunately, Alex never encountered a doctor who had even heard of his specific symptoms, and at the time it was extremely unlikely that he would have.

On the surface, Alex's feelings of dpdr came from nowhere. But persistent, ongoing pressure and stresses clearly set the stage for his shipboard mental crisis. For other people, drugs like marijuana or Ecstasy can sometimes have the same effect, with symptoms similar to what Alex described. Regarding the second interior "voice," a study of 117 individuals with DDD indicated that most (over 80%) reported no such voices at all.[9] However, a minority did experience an inner voice, a single one, best likened to an out-loud thought inside one's head, accompanied by an awareness that the voice is the person's own thoughts experienced in an intense yet disconnected fashion as a distinct "voice." This voice typically sounds like the person, is not experienced as alien, and is a commentary on the person's thoughts, feelings, or actions as if coming from a detached other, the dissociated part of the self. This infrequent experience of a "voice" in DDD distinctly differs from that of individuals with dissociative identity disorder and its variants, who often have multiple internal voices, experienced as less owned by the self and more alien, representing intrusions on the conscious self by the various alter-identities. The "voice" also differs from those of psychosis, typically experienced as coming from delusional imagined others.

These case histories and others to come have shown various manifestations of depersonalization within the context of individual lives. They by no means cover the full range of possible symptoms that can and do appear within DDD. It has taken more than a century of study for psychiatrists, psychologists, and philosophers to disseminate the symptoms described by many thousands of people. In the next chapter, we take a closer look at that historical process and its results.

2

The Path to Understanding

A Historical Exploration

The answers you get depend on the questions you ask.

—Thomas Kuhn

People suffering from depersonalization often feel they are living on the brink of insanity, or simply in some form of altered consciousness previously unknown to them. While it may be examined from many different perspectives, depersonalization/derealization disorder (DDD) is nothing new. It isn't one of many trendy acronyms making the rounds on talk shows or in social media. Feelings of depersonalization, or loss of the self, have appeared in philosophical and religious discussions for centuries (see Chapter 9). But clinically, DDD has only been observed and seriously documented in the last two centuries.

Today, the internet offers readily accessible information, but much of it is lost amid half-truths and self-styled gurus promising a cure. All too often people living with depersonalization, as well as their physicians and therapists, remain in the dark, struggling to determine what could be wrong. In years past, exhaustive searches in university or hospital libraries, or a visit with one of the few savvy psychiatrists who really knew about the condition, could reveal some answers. But even then, problems in achieving the correct diagnosis sometimes arose. Of the dozens of clinical papers that could be found, using just one could result in a wrong or misleading interpretation of the condition. For instance, among his many astute observations, Austrian psychiatrist Paul Schilder[1] is also known for the highly subjective comment that "depersonalization is the neurosis of the good looking and intelligent who want too much admiration." Taking this comment at face value and out of context would not be helpful. Visiting a clinician unfamiliar with all the

Feeling Unreal. Second Edition. Daphne Simeon and Jeffrey Abugel, Oxford University Press. © Oxford University Press 2023. DOI: 10.1093/oso/9780197622445.003.0002

literature, or at least the most relevant recently published findings, could be equally fruitless, and sometimes even harmful.

This chapter provides an overview of how the definition of DDD has evolved from the early nineteenth century to the 1970s. Through a slow stream of patient investigations, certain prevalent core symptoms of depersonalization began to emerge. Other symptoms, while as valid as they were 50 or 150 years ago, have periodically receded into the background only to resurface and receive renewed attention. Some conclusions drawn from various studies have been subject to debate or later revision by those who initially drew them. Some were downright wrong. Yet certain aspects of the disorder have been agreed upon almost universally.

We are fortunate in that depersonalization enjoys a historical record in the medical and psychological writings of Europe, beginning in France and Germany. Much of this material developed in the mid to late nineteenth century, when dramatic social changes gave rise to intellectual and philosophical explorations the world had not yet seen.

Some of the earliest clinical observations of depersonalization came from pioneering psychiatrists, sometimes referred to as "alienists" in the nineteenth century, physicians who studied the mind and assisted patients with overcoming their mental "alienation" (illness). As far back as 1838, a German doctor named Albert Zeller described five patients, all of whom "complained almost in the same terms of a lack of sensations . . . to them it was a total lack of feelings, as if they were dead . . . they claimed they could think clearly and properly about everything, but the essential was lacking even in their thoughts" (p. 525).[2]

At the same time, in France, psychiatrist Jean-Étienne Dominique Esquirol quoted patients stricken with the deep sense of melancholy known as *lypemania*: "An abyss, they say, separates them from the external world, I hear, I see, I touch . . . but I am not as formerly was. Objects do not come to me, they do not identify themselves with my being; a thick cloud, a veil changes the hue and aspects of objects" (p. 414).[3] Also in France, the alienist Eugene Billod described a patient with similar recollections: "She claimed to feel as if she were not dead or alive, as if living in a continuous dream . . . objects looked as if surrounded by a cloud; people seemed to move like shadows, and words seemed to come from a faraway world" (p. 187).[4]

Doctors observing these odd symptoms did not dismiss them as part of something more common and familiar. They began sharing information across the continent. In 1845, another German psychiatrist, Wilhelm

Griesinger (later known for his asylum reforms and efforts to integrate the mentally ill into society), shared patient accounts with Esquirol and noted: "We sometimes hear the insane, especially melancholics, complain of a quite different kind of anaesthesia . . . I see, I hear, I feel, they say but the object does not reach me; I cannot receive the sensation; it seems to me as if there was a wall between me and the external world" (p. 157).[5]

A few decades later, writings specifically dealing with depersonalization as a unique disorder emerged. In 1873, Maurice Krishaber, a Hungarian ear, nose, and throat specialist, described DDD as a possible "cérébro-cardiac" malfunction.[6] Shortly thereafter, French philosophy professor Ludovic Dugas pulled all of the anomalies exhibited by this strange condition together under the umbrella of "depersonalization" for the first time.[7] Writing with neurologist Maurice Moutier, Dugas defined depersonalization as "a state in which there is the feeling or sensation that thoughts and acts elude their self and become strange; there is an alienation of personality; in other words, a depersonalization" (p. 13).[7]

Indeed, for Dugas and Moutier, *personalization* was the normal and expected mental faculty that simply made mental events *personal*. "Personalization is the act of psychical synthesis, of appropriation or attribution of states to the self" (p. 13) they wrote.[7] Depersonalization is the dysfunction of that process. Dugas and the others were highly observant and curious, and no doubt influenced by each other, as well as by philosophers and intellectual dilettantes. Despite the differences between modern medicine and that of the nineteenth century, many of the earliest observations remain valid with few, if any, modifications, largely because what was being described by patients then is described so similarly today. Depersonalization is what it is, then and now.

Sensory Distortion Theories

As noted, records of patients suffering from "thinking without feeling,"[8] a sense of detachment, incompleteness, or total lack of feelings began accumulating in medical circles as early as the 1840s. Krishaber's observations were born out of a study of 38 patients showing a mixture of anxiety, fatigue, and depression. More than one-third of these patients complained of baffling and unpleasant mental experiences consisting of the loss of the feeling of reality.[6] Krishaber theorized that these feelings were the result of pathological changes in the body's sensory apparatus. Multiple sensory distortions would therefore lead to experiences of "self-strangeness." "One patient tells us that he feels that he is no longer himself, another that he has lost awareness of his self" (p. 171), Krishaber wrote.[6] While Dugas didn't use the term "depersonalization" until 26 years later, Krishaber's case histories marked the first true scientific study of the experience of DDD.

Another prominent theorist, Théodule Ribot, agreed with the sensory-distortion theory when he reported patients describing feelings of "being separated from the universe, or feeling as if their bodies were wrapped in an isolating substance that interposed itself between themselves and the external world; underlying these experiences there were 'physiological abnormalities whose immediate effect is to produce a change in coenesthesia'" (the general feeling of inhabiting one's body that arises from multiple integrated bodily sensations) (p. 196).[9]

In 1906, the German physician Carl Wernicke wrote about disorders of body awareness and depersonalization called *Somatopsychosen*. Citing a patient whose body had become stiff and lifeless, he noted: "She had to keep touching herself to feel the heaviness of her body. She felt as if she were dead and numb, as if it was bereft of circulation, even though she could feel her pulse and the beats of her heart. Such feelings also involved her sensory organs; she could hear but felt that her eyes were fixed to her head, and couldn't move them" (p. 242).[10]

Czech neurologist and psychiatrist Arnold Pick, after whom a type of dementia called Pick's disease was named, agreed with the sensory hypothesis. In an article, "Disorders of the Awareness of the Self," he suggested that depersonalization was accompanied by a disturbance of sensory perception.[11] Otfrid Foerster, the innovative neurologist and disciple of Wernicke, hypothesized that all sensations were composed of a specific sensory component (e.g., visual, auditory) and a corresponding muscular sensation arising from the movement itself. In healthy individuals, subjective feelings of reality and vividness resulted from the synchronized experience of these two somatic elements. In depersonalized patients, Foerster suggested, "the proprioceptive component failed to reach consciousness" (p. 14).[12] (*Proprioception* refers to the awareness of bodily sensations, position, and movement.)

These observations, along with Krishaber's sensory hypothesis, were later challenged by others like Dugas and Pierre Janet, a major figure in nineteenth-century psychology. Janet pointed out that many patients with clear sensory pathology, such as double vision (diplopia) or the loss of joint sense caused by neurosyphilis, did not complain of any sensations of un-reality, while many patients suffering from depersonalization were in fact normal from the purely sensory viewpoint.[13] Dugas wrote of a patient whose own voice sounded foreign to him: "Although he *knows* that it is his voice, *it does not give him the impression* of being his own ... Acts other than speaking are also involved ... Every time the subject moves he cannot believe that [he] is doing it himself ... The state in which the self feels that its acts are strange and beyond its control will be called here *alienation of personality* or *depersonalization*" (p. 503).[7]

Dugas' choice of words was perfect for describing the loss of "person-hood." But it was not the first time it was seen in print. The term originated in Swiss philosopher Henri Frederic Amiel's *Journal Intime*, an effusive diary in which he wrote: "All is strange to me; I am, as it were, outside my own body and individuality; I am *depersonalized*, detached, cut adrift"[14] (see Chapter 9). Now christened with proper nomenclature, depersonali-zation was for Dugas[7] a blurring of what Blaise Pascal had defined centuries before as two distinct elements of our being: "the willing mind and the au-tomaton." This blurring between the separation of the two renders all volun-tary actions automatic.

"Depersonalization behaviors not only seem automatic; to an impor-tant extent, they are," Dugas wrote. "By automatic I mean any behavior to which the self feels indifferent and foreign, and which it produces without thinking or wanting, as might happen in states of total distraction or absent mindedness" (p. 507).[7] This "apathy," a term that appears often in the litera-ture that followed, marks the emotional deadness that is one of the hallmarks of depersonalized people. It is not a decision to be indifferent or unfeeling; it is automatic and unstoppable. "Depersonalization is not a groundless illu-sion," Dugas concluded. "It is a form of apathy. Because the self is that part of the person that vibrates and feels and not what merely thinks or acts, apathy can be truly considered as the *loss of the person*" (p. 507).[7]

Memories, Real or Unreal

Nineteenth-century thinkers were also intrigued by the experience of memories. Understandably, the mystery of depersonalization emerged amid the prevalent theories about "déjà vu" phenomena (literally meaning "al-ready seen") and their opposite, "jamais vu" phenomena ("never seen").

In Germany, personal experience with DDD prompted psychiatrist Emil Kraepelin to interpret it as a dysfunction of memory relating to déjà vu: "At that moment it seems to us that all of a sudden the surroundings become hazy, as something quite remote and of no concern at all . . . The impressions from the surroundings do not convey the familiar picture of everyday reality, instead they become dream-like or shadowy . . . as if seen through a veil" (p. 410).[15]

Dugas initially regarded the presence of depersonalization as evidence for the view that déjà vu was a form of "double consciousness," a popular term of the era used to describe dual or alternating personalities. But he changed his mind completely when he took a closer look at depersonalization all by itself.

Still, the compelling similarities between strange phenomena like hypnotic suggestion, dreaming, déjà vu, jamais vu, and depersonalization kept these mysterious mind states swimming together in the same fishbowl, so to speak, as observers watched, took notes, and tried to determine their possible connection. But all along, they sensed that there was something singular and different about depersonalization.

Hollow Selves

At an 1880 meeting with peers in Berlin, psychiatrist O. Shafer shared his observations of patients with what he considered a subtype of melancholia that he called *Melancholia Anaesthetica*: "When these patients complain of their suffering, they relate it explicitly to an emptiness, hollowness in their head, or in the pit of their stomach; of a discomfort of not reaching the surroundings with their inner selves . . . [Patients] have lost the feeling of activity or effort that used to accompany their thoughts and actions, and so they feel in themselves like lifeless machines" (p. 242).[16]

Gustave Wilhelm Störring, a psychiatrist who turned to philosophy later in life, believed that "coenesthesia" lay at the heart of *self-experiencing*. He argued that "organic sensations are a condition of consciousness of self; and the awareness of one's body, which is due to them, must be regarded as one constituent of it" (p. 290).[17] Hence, disturbed perception played a role in the genesis of self-strangeness. Coenesthesia, lack of activity-feelings, and power of perception were all involved in an altered experience of the self, Störring theorized.[17]

A fellow German psychiatrist, Max Lowy, modified Störring's ideas by fine-tuning the concept of activity-feelings to one of "action-feelings." This referred to a conscious mental representation of the experience of "what it feels like to carry out a particular mental activity (including perception), rather than to accompanying emotional feelings like pleasure or dislike" (p. 460).[18] For instance, during recollection of personal memories, there is, in addition to the information retrieved, a distinct sense of what it feels like to remember something, a *feeling* of delving into the past. Lowy wrote, "The action-feeling of psychological activity, or thought-feeling; it normally accompanies every psychological act, it provides altogether the awareness of the reality of perceived objects . . . in its absence colours and tones become distant and strange, things become unreal, as if from another world."[18]

Janet, who as noted earlier challenged the sensory distortion theory, is also well known for introducing the words "dissociation" and "subconscious" into psychology's terminology. He attributed the nineteenth-century affliction "hysteria" (later known as "conversion disorder," in which a psychological conflict manifests itself in the form of some bodily dysfunction such as hysterical paralysis or blindness) to imbalances in "psychic energy" and "psychic tension" (the use of the word "psychic" simply means psychological, relating to the mind). Janet considered depersonalization to be a manifestation of "psychasthenia," an antiquated term for any nonspecific condition marked by phobias, obsessions, compulsions, or excessive anxiety (p. 318).[19]

Certainly, these mental anomalies often accompany depersonalization or mark the beginnings of it. But Janet also stressed the presence of a *sentiment d'incompletude*, an experience of incompleteness that many observers found well represented in Dugas' source for the term "depersonalization," Amiel's *Journal Intime*.[14] "What characterizes the feeling of depersonalization . . . is that the patient perceives himself as an incomplete, unachieved person," Janet stated.[13] This feeling of being incomplete is indeed a core part of the experience of depersonalization, in terms of one's being out of sync with one's "normal" self-experience. It can also be a secondary feeling, referring to reflections of what the self and life "used to be" or "might have been" that can emerge in people who have been depersonalized for a long time. As we will see in Chapter 9, Amiel's journal graphically depicts both these attitudes.

Overall, however, Janet's theories brought about a major shift in the predominant thinking on depersonalization. Janet believed that all psychic activity was either primary or secondary. Primary psychic activity encompassed everything that was evoked by external stimuli—from knee jerks to memories. Secondary psychic activity was a background echo elicited by representations of primary acts. By conferring upon primary experiences a feeling of vividness (*l'impression de vie*), this secondary echo creates the illusion of a continuous flow of psychic activity: "Thousands of resonances, constituted by secondary actions, fill the spirit during the intervals between external stimuli, and give the impression that it is never empty" (p. 126).[19] Disconnection between these primary and secondary psychic processes could result in depersonalization-like symptoms, connoting a self not experienced as continuous. Janet's language was different, but his theory remains surprisingly contemporary.

From the Psychological to the Biological

As the twentieth century emerged, existing theories about depersonalization still seemed inadequate because there were simply too many aspects of the condition that remained unexplained. Depersonalization began to be viewed in terms of the loss of some brain mechanism that causes the *feeling* of mental experiences and attribution to the self as the agent who experiences them— the sense that "my experiences are mine," commonly referred to as agency.

In the 1930s, Heidelberg psychiatrist Wilhelm Mayer-Gross's now-famous paper "On Depersonalization" reviewed the theories, case histories, and speculations up to that time, in an attempt to elucidate the nature of the disorder.[20] Mayer-Gross was first to highlight the distinction between depersonalization and derealization, two manifestations of what is now considered the same disorder of DDD. Much of what Mayer-Gross said was referenced again and again by other writers in succeeding decades, up to the present.

Mayer-Gross believed that depersonalization was an expression of a "pre-formed functional response" of the brain, analogous to delirium, catatonia, or seizures. He took exception to theorists who focused on isolated symptoms of the disorder, such as increased self-observation, loss of emotional response, or impairment of memory: "It is a characteristic form of reaction of the central organ, which can be set going by different causes. . . . The difficulty of description by means of normal speech, the defiance of comparison, the persistence of the syndrome in the face of complete insight into its paradoxical nature—all these point to something more than purely psychic connections. Such a disturbance cannot be explained by the loss of a little wheel out of the clockwork" (p. 118).[20]

Mayer-Gross recorded another important observation, which holds particularly true for people who can remember the exact moment of onset of their depersonalization, especially when the trigger was marijuana or some other substance: "Depersonalization and derealization often appear suddenly, without any warning. A patient sitting quietly reading by the fireside is overwhelmed by it in a full blast together with an acute anxiety attack. In some cases it disappears for a short period, only to reappear and finally persist" (p. 118).[20]

This sudden psychic blast from seemingly nowhere has appeared not only in the annals of medicine, but in literature and philosophy as well. Years before Mayer-Gross's 1935 account, there was a description of a similar type of panic onset in William James's classic work, *The Varieties of Religious Experiences*, published in 1902. In the chapter entitled "The Sick Soul," James relays the words of a French writer who has captured the flavor of the kind of panic that can sometimes trigger chronic depersonalization:

> I went one evening into a dressing room in the twilight to procure some article that was there, suddenly there fell upon me without any warning, just as if it came out of the darkness, a horrible fear of my own existence. Simultaneously there arose in my mind the image of an epileptic patient whom I had seen in the asylum, a black-haired youth with greenish skin, entirely idiotic, who used to sit all day on one of the benches, or rather shelves against the wall, with his knees drawn up against his chin, and the coarse gray undershirt, which was his only garment, drawn over them enclosing his entire figure. . . . This image and my fear entered into a species of combination with each other. That shape am I, I felt, potentially. Nothing that I possess can defend me against that fate, if the hour for it should strike for me as it struck for him. There was such a horror of him, and such a perception of my own merely momentary discrepancy from him, that it was as if something hitherto solid within my breast gave way entirely, and I became a mass of quivering fear. After this the universe was changed for me altogether.[21]

For some people, William James is describing with uncanny precision the moment that marked the onset of their own depersonalization. The inexplicable panic that he is attempting to explain goes well beyond the clichéd images of sweaty palms and rapid heartbeat associated with panic or anxiety attacks—the certainty of imminent insanity that, unbeknownst to the victim, will pass after the attack lies at its heart. While James does not tell us what happened to this particular person, the inclusion of this experience in "The Sick Soul" seems particularly appropriate. Depersonalized people, who sometimes say they have "lost their soul," may well recall a single episode like this as the very moment when their soul departed. Of course, others can experience this kind of incident once, or repeatedly, without the end result of chronic depersonalization.

James refers more specifically to feelings of depersonalization and unreality in the chapter titled "The Reality of the Unseen," where he writes: "Like all positive affections of consciousness, the sense of reality has its negative counterpart in the shape of a feeling of unreality by which persons may be haunted, and of which one sometimes hears complaint." Drawing from other sources, he then quotes the French poet Louise Ackermann, who wrote in *Pensées d'un Solitaire*: "When I see myself surrounded by beings as ephemeral and incomprehensible as I am myself, and all excitedly pursuing pure chimeras, I experience a strange feeling of being in a dream. It seems to me as if I have loved and suffered and that erelong I shall die, in a dream. My last word will be, 'I have been dreaming.'" This sense of the unreality of things, James comments, "may become a carking [perplexing] pain, and even lead to suicide."[21]

James the psychologist does not suggest any treatment for the condition he explored only briefly, while Mayer-Gross, ultimately convinced that depersonalization was founded in some cerebral dysfunction, did not see a lot of point in psychologically minded attempts to treat the condition: "Writers make abundant use of hypotheses about narcissism, libido-cathexis, etc.," he wrote. "I have found it difficult to gain any fruitful idea from such suggestions or from the suggestions of psychoanalytic writers about depersonalization. The disagreement between them is rather discouraging" (p. 118).[20] This did not discourage psychologists from continuing to propose new theories for decades. But Mayer-Gross concluded that depersonalization should be regarded as a physiological disorder, summed up by his well-known phrase of a "non-specific pre-formed functional response of the brain."[20]

While in some ways Mayer-Gross's assessment of depersonalization has stood the test of time, especially when it comes to the acute automated depersonalization that accompanies life-threatening or near-death experiences, today's thinking draws from both physiological and psychological explanations, with a fresh understanding of the fact that they are not incompatible with one another—the brain and the mind are not separable.

Psychoanalytic Theories

Psychoanalytic thinkers have formulated their own theories about the origins of depersonalization for many decades, dating back to Freud. Most of these writers have agreed on one point: depersonalization serves as a psychological defensive strategy ("defense mechanism" in stricter psychoanalytic lingo) of some sort. However, what depersonalization might be defending against can vary greatly from person to person; hence the diversity and richness of these theories, which can accommodate differing psychologies in different individuals—we are not all the same. Clearly, a lot of thought has gone into trying to figure out the psychological processes underpinning what many people, including physicians, have long perceived as an obscure condition, or merely as a part of some other disorder.

As we touched upon in Chapter 1, Freud had something to say about the condition after he had experienced intense though fleeting derealization while he first saw the Acropolis in 1904, up close and in person. As he later analyzed his experience at 80 years of age, in the now-famous letter to Romain Rolland "A Disturbance of Memory on the Acropolis" Freud wrote: "These derealizations are remarkable phenomena which are still little understood . . . These phenomena are to be observed in two forms: the subject feels either that a piece of reality or that a piece of his own self is strange to him. In the latter case we speak of 'depersonalizations'; derealizations and depersonalizations are intimately connected."[22] "Their positive counterparts," Freud added, "are known as *fausse reconnaissance, déjà vu, déjà raconte* etc., illusions in which we seek to accept something as belonging to our ego, just as in the derealizations we are anxious to keep something out of us."[22] According to Freud, "naively mystical" and non-psychological attempts to explain déjà vu phenomena interpret them as evidence of a former life. "Depersonalization leads us on to the extraordinary condition of '*double conscience*' which is more correctly described at 'split personality'" (p. 245).[22]

Freud also referred to the defensive characteristics of depersonalization and derealization in his famous case history that came to be known as the "Wolf Man."[23] Considered one of Freud's most complex and detailed accounts of the psychotherapeutic process, the subject of the story was a wealthy young Russian who sought Freud's help because he felt that there was a "veil" between himself and the real world. This was coupled with intense fear of wolves, specifically the fear of being eaten by them. While little is told of his specific symptoms, the mention of the "veil" indeed sounds like derealization. The case centers around a dream the man had as a child, of white wolves perched in a tree and staring at him as he looked out through an open window. The man's early childhood was rich with material for his doctor to explore. He had either actually or in his imagination seen his parents having sex, thus witnessing the "primal scene"; he had been sexually abused by his older sister, who had fondled his genitals; and furthermore the sister, aware of his wolf phobia, had tormented him by periodically surprising him with pictures of the animals.

Freud's lengthy analysis dissected each of these and other events that happened to the young Russian before the age of five. Probing the man's memories deeply and methodically, Freud was able to build his case for "infantile neurosis," centering on the oedipal conflict and its unsuccessful resolution. In his early life, the Wolf Man had experienced libidinal conflicts that remained unresolved, resulting in persistent neurotic guilt and fear of retaliation in the form of the wolves. Even in Freud's time, the centrality of the oedipal theory was being challenged by analysts like Adler, Jung, and Janet. Contemporary analysts may be more struck by the more "real" traumas in Wolf Man's early life (sister), rather than his intrapsychic oedipal conflict (primal scene), and might conceptualize the Wolf Man's derealization as a chronic manifestation of unresolved early trauma. In the end, the young Russian apparently recovered, in part through Freud's analysis of his unconscious conflicts and in part, as Freud himself noted, because his fortunes and family were lost after the Russian Revolution of 1917, assuaging his long-endured feelings of neurotic guilt—"real" punishment helped Wolf Man's unreality.

Ultimately, Freud knew that there was much to be explored in depersonalization/derealization. He interpreted his own intense derealization before the Acropolis as his mind's defense against the guilt he himself felt about succeeding in life so far beyond his own father, who had died in obscurity. While Freud's writings on depersonalization specifically were limited, his 1919 essay devoted to the "uncanny" (*Das Unheimliche*) captures a fundamental duality and ambiguity: *heimlich* refers to the familiar but also, secondarily, to the concealed, and *unheimlich* is therefore both its opposite and its equivalent.[24]

Founded on this tension between the familiar and the hidden, *uncanniness* challenges the validity of the familiar and renders it unreal.

Freud's followers attempted to explain the condition within the context of his theories, specifically the tripartite structural theory of the mind, which divides the psyche into three parts: id, ego, and superego. Ego is the reality-oriented part of the mind, the mediator and compromiser between the instinctual and primitive id, which contains all our drives like sexuality and aggression, and the superego, the seat of our moral conscience.

Several theorists thus attempted to understand the psychology of depersonalization focusing on drive theory and the vicissitudes of the ego. Austrian psychologist Paul Federn viewed the ego as a "homogeneous structure, which is characterized by a specific ego feeling and an ego experience" (p. 235).[25] Accordingly, depersonalization and derealization were disturbances of the ego caused by a *lack* of libidinal investment affecting the "ego structural core" and the "ego boundaries," respectively, and resulting in unreality of self-experience.[25] Psychiatrist Clarence Paul Oberndorf, who wrote several papers on depersonalization during the 1930s, proposed a model in part opposite to Federn's, theorizing that an *increased* libidinal investment in thought processes was central to depersonalization[26]—he was referring to the hypertrophied overthinking encountered in many with DDD.

Later, in the 1950s, Oberndorf further conceptualized depersonalization as a defensive process against anxiety-producing intrapsychic conflicts.[27] Although there was no single generally accepted theory among traditional psychodynamic authors, most did conceptualize depersonalization as an unconscious defensive maneuver against unresolved and overwhelming feelings, experiences, and conflicts, wherein more adaptive defense mechanisms have failed. "Defense mechanism" is yet another tricky term whose meaning has evolved over the decades. Where dissociation is concerned, contemporary theorists would agree that dissociation is more than a defense mechanism (i.e., a largely unconscious way of processing internal conflict); it is a subjectively experienced state-of-mind or self-state. Nonetheless, such as a state of being can clearly serve defensive purposes.

Sometimes, formulations made in the older psychoanalytic literature (we visit more contemporary analytic perspectives in Chapter 13) ring true to a depersonalized individual who may encounter them in their search for answers or upon a visit to a psychotherapist. Some of these commentaries are more dated than others yet remain part of the evolution of psychoanalytic thinking about the condition, and subject to interpretation through more modern lenses. For instance, Paul Schilder, in a well-known paper on the treatment of depersonalization, wrote: "I am inclined to stress the fact that the patient with depersonalization has been admired very much by the parents for his intellectual and physical gifts. A great amount of admiration and erotic interest has been spent upon the child. He expects that this erotic inflow should be continuous. The final outcome of such an attitude by the parents will not be different from the outcome of an attitude of neglect."[28]

In its original terms, this formulation may appear stiff and antiquated, but translated into more contemporary language it has much more to offer. Schilder goes on to say that the parental attitude of considering the child a "showpiece" rather than a complete human being eventually results in deep dissatisfaction. Initial self-adulation, stemming from an identification with parental attitudes, will ultimately be followed by emotional emptiness, even though intellect remains intact and the person may appear quite normal or even successful to others. Schilder is, in fact, simply talking about the inevitable emotional neglect of children raised as narcissistic extensions of parents, the trials and tribulations of self-esteem formation in such scenarios, and the very detrimental impact on the development of a healthy self—a person who was never known to others may never truly know himself, but instead feeds on the admiration of others.

Schilder also had something to say about the self-scrutinizing component of depersonalization: "All depersonalized patients observe themselves continuously and with great zeal; they compare their present dividedness-within-themselves with their previous oneness-with-themselves. Self-observation is compulsive with these patients. The tendency to self-observation continuously rejects the tendency to live."[28] This is a common phenomenon in depersonalized patients, and the compulsive self-observation can be viewed as a defense again truly experiencing and living, when these are too overwhelming and risky to undertake. Schilder also made some astute observations about the "automaton" aspects of depersonalization, which he called *negation of experiencing*:

> In clear cut cases, the patients complain that they no longer have an ego, but are mechanisms, automatons, puppets—what they do seems not done by them, but happens automatically . . . raw materials of their somatic [body] sensations are unchanged. . . . Their lack of memory images is not a loss of imagery, but rather an inhibition of existing memories. Such patients fight, defend themselves against their perceptions; they negate internally their

entire experience, and prevent themselves from experiencing anything fully.[28]

In the above observation, Schilder is proposing that the hypoemotionality of depersonalization is not a deficit but rather a defense, an inhibition of memories that for whatever reasons are too painful and overwhelming to emotionally recall. Nonetheless, many patients may remain capable of complex achievements, which, however, are experienced as fake and without deeper meaning—part of a false, showpiece self. In fact, some depersonalized patients do make reference to themselves as "fake" or as "imposters."

Other psychologists, before and after Schilder, either concurred with his views, put their own spin on existing ego psychology theories, or forged new ones. Fritz Wittels, in 1940, saw depersonalization as resulting from identification with a large number of phantom images (unintegrated identifications), the ego being unable to accept any one of them as the real self, due to superego condemnation of each of them.[29] Along similar lines, psychologist Edith Jacobson became interested in depersonalization after studying female prisoners who depersonalized in response to being imprisoned by the Nazis in World War II. In a 1959 commentary, she stated that depersonalization always represents an attempt to solve a narcissistic conflict, and she viewed depersonalization as a struggle between conflicting identifications. Unacceptable identifications are defended against by disowning and denying those undesirable parts of the self, and these shifts between the various conflicting identifications produce feelings of depersonalization.[30]

Similarly, another psychoanalyst, C. N. Sarlin, also conceptualized depersonalization as defending against conflicting ego identifications. The disorder may occur, he said, when a conflict between the individual's mother and father becomes internalized as two conflicting aspects of the child's ego. The struggle between simultaneous hostile identifications with both parents may cause the individual to lose his or her identity.[31]

Jacob Arlow, a well-known ego psychology theorist, agreed with the thinking that depersonalization represents the outcome of intrapsychic conflict "in which the ego utilizes, in a more or less successful way, various defenses against anxiety. The split in the ego which results in the dissociation between the *experiencing* self and the *observing* self takes place in the interest of defense."[32] Depersonalization, he believed, boils down to a specific set of reactions of the ego in the face of great danger, real or imagined. The danger is experienced as pertinent to the participating self and can thus be distanced from the observing self. Arlow, who also wrote about déjà vu and distortions in the sense of time, said in the 1960s that depersonalization and derealization represent a "dissociation of the function of immediate experience from the function of self-observation."[32]

Arlow took the view that the essential ego alternation in depersonalization is a dissociation of two ego functions that are normally integrated: the function of self-observation and the function of experiencing and participating. Normally, both functions occur alongside and are more or less integrated, often seamlessly. In depersonalization, he pointed out, the participating self is partially, though not completely, repudiated; the patient is still able to maintain some sense of connection and some feeling of identification. Simply put, people with DDD are inclined to observe, rather than experience, the self.

Arlow was one of the few psychoanalysts to bring up the similarities between dreaming and depersonalization. Indeed, feeling as if in a dream is one of the more common complaints among depersonalized patients. Two characteristics of depersonalization, feelings of unreality and the split of the sense of self into an observing self and a participating self, are prominent in dreaming. "Usual" dreaming is all participating self—the observing self is suspended in sleep. But in lucid dreaming, both self-functions are operating (learning to lucid dream is a therapeutic technique for nightmares!). Lucid dreaming is an altered state of consciousness, rare or unattainable for many people ("Snap out of it, it's a dream," says the observing to the participating self in sleep). Depersonalization may be something akin to lucid dreaming, where the two functions of participating and observing are split.

The well-known German-Swiss psychiatrist turned philosopher Karl Jaspers defined DDD in terms of the "I" quality, the sense of ownership accompanying perceptions, memories, thoughts, or bodily sensations, resulting in *personalization*. "If these psychic manifestations are accompanied by the awareness that they are not mine, but are alien, automatic, independent, arriving from elsewhere, they are called *depersonalization*" (p. 121).[33] Here we are exiting the more abstract domain of the "ego" and entering the more commonsensical domain of self and personhood. Ego and self partly overlap but are not the same—a simply put distinction is that the ego contains conscious awareness, whereas the self includes the ego but extends to one's entire being and experience.

All these psychological theories followed Mayer-Gross's 1935 statement that such theories were devoid of any fruitful ideas. Certainly, the person who can trace his or her onset of depersonalization to a specific event seemingly devoid of meaningful psychological content (e.g., "I smoked pot, end of story") might not at first be interested in the possibility of deeply rooted psychological causes. Alternatively, excessive conviction about a seemingly "obvious" psychological cause, or no cause at all for that matter, can obscure more subtle, enduring, and powerful dynamics that might eventually trigger the onset of DDD. In this light, a person's initial conviction that their depersonalization is not driven by complex psychological processes should never be taken at face value.

Altered Sense of Time

Distortion of time perception is a frequent complaint of depersonalized individuals; it is often mentioned today on depersonalization-themed websites and in personal stories. In a 1946 paper ("The Depersonalization Syndrome") H. J. Shorvon reviewed aspects of his study of 66 patients. One-third of them complained of changes in time perception. Shorvon cited a statement by Aubrey Lewis that time consciousness "is an aspect of all conscious activity; it is essential to all reality. In *déjà vu* there is a brief inability to actualize the present, which in consequence is projected into the past."[34] Of time disturbance in depersonalization, again Shorvon quoted Lewis, who said:

> They [time disturbances] illustrate many of the outstanding features of the disorder; the inability to evoke the past readily or clearly, to distinguish the present from the past or future; there is paradoxically the increased quickness with which time passes though it seems to drag along, the seeming remoteness of the recent past, the unconfirmed feeling of the inability to judge the length of time.[34]

Paul Schilder adds that "the present is a concept which has meaning only in relation to experiencing personalities. The inanimate has no past, present or future. . . . Cases of depersonalization, whose total experience is splintered, all have an altered perception of time. In extreme cases, time seems to them to be at a standstill, or the present seems to be like the distant past" (p. 310).[28]

"The only reason for time is so that everything doesn't happen at once," said Albert Einstein in his disarmingly understated way. Yet to depersonalized people, time often does not unfold in the normal manner; past, present, and future can seem indistinguishable.

Obsessiveness

The obsessional aspects of depersonalization have not been ignored through the years, though Sir Martin Roth in 1960 perceptively pointed out the major difference between obsessional states such as contemporary obsessive-compulsive disorder, and the kind of obsessiveness present in depersonalization. Roth identified a particular subgroup among depersonalized individuals that included patients fraught with ongoing free-floating anxiety and excessive rumination. He proposed what he called the "phobic-anxiety-depersonalization syndrome" (PADS), with core symptoms of agoraphobia and depersonalization. Depersonalization, in any context, does not involve classic obsessive rituals, like hand washing, or outwardly eccentric compulsive behavior. Roth remarked: "Obsessional features commonly present, though rarely in the forefront of the picture, are a compulsive self-scrutiny and preoccupations with fears of disease, insanity or loss of self-control."[35]

Roth also pointed out the distinction between DDD and classic phobias, which involve specific fears like flying, or heights, or creatures such as snakes and spiders: "The free-floating anxiety which is said to be characteristic of anxiety neurosis proper, is very common in the phobic-anxiety-depersonalization state," Roth observed.[35] But these patients are unable to suppress their anxiety altogether by avoiding feared objects or situations in the way a person with a phobia might. If the center of the fear is the self, or existence itself, escape or avoidance is impossible.

Years later, as PADS came to be looked at as more of an anxiety disorder, Roth revised his thinking, stating that "it is plain that depersonalization was given an undeserved prominence in the original description."[36] Like Mayer-Gross, Roth later viewed depersonalization as a pre-formed brain response shaped by evolution: "Depersonalization comprises a state of heightened arousal together with dissociation of emotion and thus serves as an adaptive mechanism which enhances the chances of survival in acute danger," he wrote.[36]

The obsessional components of depersonalization were further explored by psychiatrist Evan Torch, who observed that there is a particular type of patient whose obsession is observing himself or his "vegetative functions."

Torch wrote, "Even in a typical case of hypochondria, conversion neurosis or depression, *in the background of an obsessional personality* it is not hard to see how continual, repetitive preoccupation with one's self can lead to a feeling of unreality, based in no small way on the fact that even to a philosopher . . . the question of just where to locate centrality of 'self' or 'being' is an uncomfortable one to face."[37] No wonder philosophers live in their own separate world, for many of us—they think too much.

Among patients with DDD, Torch, like Roth, also noticed a particular subtype of the disorder, which he called the "intellectual-obsessive depersonalization syndrome." This subcategory, Torch said, is composed of a complex combination of alternating states of depersonalization and obsessive self-scrutiny. The end result is the "burned out" depersonalization patient, who, although still fully in touch with reality, refuses to acknowledge its intrinsic meaning.[37]

Viewing One's Self

One of the many intriguing metaphors used by depersonalized people is that they feel as if they are viewing themselves, as if watching a movie. Depersonalization involves an unpleasant sense of self-observation, an exaggerated hyperawareness of one's mental (and even bodily) processes. The split between the observing and the acting self (see Arlow earlier) can, at its most extreme, become an out-of-body experience, although for most people with DDD it is not common. Noyes and colleagues explored this split when discussing partial or complete depersonalization among accident victims. For the 66% of the "normal" individuals who suddenly depersonalized, the condition appeared to be "an adaptive mechanism that combines opposing reaction tendencies, the one serving to intensify alertness and the other to dampen potentially disorganizing emotion" (p. 376).[38]

William James eloquently captured the process that gone awry can lead to one part of the self viewing the other:

> Whatever I may be thinking of, I am always at the same time more or less aware of myself, of my personal existence. At the same time it is I who am aware; so that the total self of me, being as it were duplex, partly known and partly knower, partly object and partly subject, must have two aspects discriminated in it, of which for shortness we may call one the Me and the

other the I. I call these "discriminated aspects," and not separate things, because the identity of I and Me even in the very act of their discrimination, is
perhaps the most ineradicable dictum of common-sense.[39]

When this I/Me or subject/object dichotomy that James is describing, normally seamlessly integrated and minimally in our conscious awareness or
outside of it, becomes split, then the experience of the self, which contains
both, is one of depersonalization.

Social Factors

Depersonalization means different things to different cultures. In Western
culture, we may be witnessing a rise in DDD, possibly attributable to the
widespread use of illicit recreational drugs, the intense isolation of the
COVID-19 pandemic, and the increased reliance on remote technology
for communication. But the question also arises as to whether modern
society is, in itself, a cause of depersonalization. Writing about depersonalization and its relation to society in the 1970s, James and Jane Cattell
said, "People working under centralized bureaucracies are routinized,
humiliated, and thereby dehumanized. The economic systems prevent involvement and foster detachment. It [sic] generates competition, creates
feelings of inadequacy and fear of human obsolescence. It creates hostility
and suspiciousness."[40]

Quoting the French writer Simone de Beauvoir, Cattell and Cattell agreed
that the basic characteristic of the American value orientation is that the
source of one's value and truth is perceived in things and not in oneself.
Consequently, material comfort has a high place in the value hierarchy.
Success puts its emphasis on rewards. "The success system, which William
James has colorfully described as 'the bitch Goddess success,' is comprised
[sic] of money, prestige, power and security."[40]

For many people, the safest road to success lies within the embrace of a
corporation, usually the bigger the better. Corporations bind their employees
through job security, wage scales, health insurance, sick leave, and retirement
plans, making it difficult to leave no matter how dehumanizing a particular
job may become. Such perks are especially attractive to individuals who try
their hand at their own enterprise and fail. The desire for security is particularly strong in those who have taken risks and lost.

The impact of bureaucratization is a movement from an "inner-directed" individual to "other-directed" individual, Cattell and Cattell suggest, characterized by (1) orientation toward situational rather than internalized goals; (2) extreme sensitivity to the opinions of others; (3) excessive need for approval; (4) conformity on internal experience as well as on externals; (5) loss of achievement orientation; and (6) loss of individualism. The clear ramifications are that if one defines oneself in terms of occupation or works purely for increased wealth and social status, the loss of a job or a sudden social change could easily result in alienation and the loss of a sense of self. The self had been rooted in shallow ground to begin with.

Some of Cattell and Cattell's observations may now seem out of date. Certainly, more people are able to work independently today, even if they have to invest a few years of conformity to corporate life in order to gain experience. People change jobs and locations far more often as well. But other factors of today's society may contribute to an altered sense of the self and its place in society in other ways. The post-9/11 world is increasingly insecure. People were incredulous when they viewed the Twin Towers collapsing on live television and, in an unprecedented way, real life "seemed like a movie" to the national consciousness. Certainly, our shared sense of security, and reality, was shaken as never before. Still, these experiences could more broadly be classified as experiences of modern-day "alienation" and may or may not bear directly on the clinical syndrome of depersonalization.

Evidence reveals depersonalization did in fact emerge profoundly during the COVID pandemic of 2020 and beyond, as social distancing and isolation wreaked havoc with familiar, safe, day-to-day routines. This rang particularly true when it came to internet use as our primary social connection, and brought internet addiction to the forefront in an unprecedented manner. Today's cyberculture may also contribute to a blurring of reality, particularly in young people who, spending countless hours in cyberspace, have learned how easy it is to be anyone at any time while online (see Chapter 14).

Early Family Influences

Cattell and Cattell, and other writers on the subject, believe that the self is largely a product of culture, in that the individual picks up reactions of others and incorporates them into a meaningful, coherent self-structure. The true self begins at home, where in infancy having an attentive primary caretaker fosters basic trust and security in the child, who begins to recognize itself as a distinct being through the recognition by others. So what processes can bring about a miscarriage in identity development, leading to depersonalization? Distorted messages, mixed messages, or non-messages, and the relationships of the individual's perceptions of these messages to his or her emerging concept of self and the world are particularly relevant, according to Cattell and Cattell. "To the extent that there is a disturbance in the normal separation-individuation phase of development (sense of autonomy), the perception of the mother is distorted and, therefore, perception of the self is distorted. Thus, there is interference with reality contact—difficulty in distinguishing between self and objects."[40]

An example Cattell and Cattell cite is artificial feeding times, which prevent the infant from feeling that its desires and actions will result in being fed. The psychological impacts of regimented and forced feeding were elaborated by Austrian psychologist Bruno Bettelheim, known for his work with disturbed children: "When we feel that we cannot influence the important things that happen to us but that they follow the dictates of some inexorable power, then we give up trying to learn how to act or change them."[41] When development miscarries in this manner, the self can split into two parts, the "true" self and the "false" self, or the "subject" and the "object."

Cattell and Cattell elaborate that the true self is the unembodied self that functions as observer, controller, and critic of what the body is experiencing and doing. The true self translates into action what one wants to be. Only the true self feels real. The false self, in contrast, is built on compliance and subjugation, molded by the intentions and expectations of significant others or what one imagines these to be. The body is perceived more as an object among other objects in the world than as the alive core of one's individual being. The individual feels that he or she is a spectator of what the body is doing rather than a participant-observer. In the words of Scottish psychologist R. D. Laing, describing the divided self, "The false, conforming, outer self had arisen in childhood, in compliance with the intentions and expectations of the parents or with what one imagines to be their intentions and expectations. The true self, with its genuine feelings, had meanwhile retreated in fear, detaching itself from the actions of the false self that seemed like betrayals."[42] Cattell and Cattell summarized that vulnerability to depersonalization comes about through deficiencies and distortions of the patient's experiences with nurturance in infancy and in subsequent stages of personality development. These include exposure to double-bind messages, rejection of the true self, and fostering of the development of the false self. In essence, the infant is programmed to deny satisfaction of its needs and expression of its emotions in order to avoid extreme anxiety. Such repudiation leads to repression of unacceptable needs and emotions that are not consciously recognized. This is the intrapsychic programming that must be dealt with in treatment.

Though Cattell and Cattell's astute observations date back several decades, they are very contemporary, though the lingo has changed. Though our historical overview of DDD ends here, with the 1970s, the ensuing 50 years have greatly broadened and deepened our understanding of how psychopathology can develop from very early in life—reflected in the fields of childhood trauma and attachment theory, the work of infant researchers, as well as intersubjective and relational theories of mind emphasizing the role of mutuality, recognition, and mentalization in healthy early development (see Chapters 7 and 13).

3

Symptoms and Scales

The finest words in the world are only vain sounds if you cannot understand them

—Anatole France

Understanding the Language

People suffering from depersonalization and derealization (dpdr) may be quite adept at communicating with each other about their dissociative experiences. While certain words and phrases are immediately recognizable to them, what they are attempting to describe may seem nothing less than odd or crazy to friends, family, or even clinicians. It is, then, very important to be able to reliably identify "catch phrases" that typically emerge during the diagnostic evaluation of a person who potentially presents with depersonalization/derealization disorder (DDD).

Some cultures have many different words to describe the subtle variations of a single concept, experience, or phenomenon. The Inuit language's multitude of sounds to signify "snow" is the classic example, understandably so considering the snowy climates where it is spoken. The vast terrain of unreality would benefit from a broader lexicon to help find words for the unspeakable. To communicate their condition, depersonalized people must rely on the subtle nuances of simpler words or phrases often used as metaphor to capture the experiential with language. The word *unreal* is *the* keyword for depersonalized people. To describe it, they must often use metaphors that may be more understandable to others.

Catch phrases can be misinterpreted, and often are. An expression like "I feel nothing" could easily be attributed to depression, or even to negative symptoms of schizophrenia. "I feel detached" may sound like an intellectual or philosophical complaint, a general sense of alienation rather than a subjective state of consciousness. Concerned listeners may even wonder if the term *unreal* means the same as *not real*.

Feeling Unreal. Second Edition. Daphne Simeon and Jeffrey Abugel, Oxford University Press. © Oxford University Press 2023. DOI: 10.1093/oso/9780197622445.003.0003

An article by Filip and Susanna Radovic, published in 2002 in the journal *Philosophy, Psychiatry, and Psychology,* explored some of the terminology used by depersonalized patients, including the term *unreal.*[1] Considering the broadness and prevalence of the word *unreal* in our culture, people often use the expression "unreal" without connoting an underlying dpdr experience, the authors point out—rather, they are talking about something way out of the ordinary. Life seems *unreal* to someone who is depersonalized, yet it also may seem *unreal* to someone who has just won the lottery. The latter person may be having an intellectual or emotional experience of unreality, like in "this cannot be happening to me," because of their "unbelievable" good fortune. Alternatively, they may in fact be experiencing a short-lived bout of genuine dpdr, essentially for the very same reason, triggered by the overwhelmingness of the extreme event. According to the Radovics, in everyday language the term *unreal* has three primary usages:

1. Not existing (as in the case of a mythological being)
2. Fake, made up, or artificial (such as a toy stuffed animal)
3. Not normative, typical, or optimal (as in "he is not a real [i.e., a true] friend")

When depersonalized people say "life feels unreal," their meaning can involve any or all three of these usages. Ultimately, however, the experiential shift of dpdr goes beyond what is meant by any of the above definitions. The authors liken this change to that of a dream state—it cannot be described satisfactorily within the existent *real* and *unreal* parameters. You may know (after having it and upon awakening) that a dream is not real, but it can *feel* very real while dreaming—dreaming is an altered state of consciousness, like depersonalization.

"Dreams are often accompanied by a varying degree of a sense of reality (or unreality) that has no obvious correlation with the amount of strangeness or atypicality present in the dream," the Radovics explain. "This particular feeling of unreality may be a salient and distinct feature of a dream and is often reported by subjects after awakening" (p. 276).[1] This point about dreams is particularly interesting because many depersonalized people describe their state as "dream-like," yet any relationships between dreaming and dpdr remain unexplored; anecdotally, when sharing their dreams, DDD patients may mention that they felt depersonalized, or not, within a dream.

The "as if" nature of dpdr experiences also comes into play. Words like *mechanical, dead,* or *lifeless* enter the picture, as well as the use of metaphors such as "I feel *like* a robot." Such descriptions reflect how difficult it can be to capture dpdr with a literal vocabulary. The only way to give an approximate account of one's subjective experiences is then to paint a picture in words. The "as if" prefix reflects the uncertainty about the adequacy of a proposed description—it is the best verbalization a patient can come up with. There is a second important aspect to the "as if" qualifier, reflecting that a patient is not psychotic or delusional—despite having dpdr, reality testing remains intact. The patient does *not* believe that they *are* a robot, but rather it *feels as if* they are functioning like one.

The word *feel* is also fraught with its own mysteries. A person may suffer immensely from lack of feeling when hypoemotionality and numbing comprise one of their core depersonalization symptoms, yet suffering itself is a feeling—a negative one, a pained state of mind. But suffering alone is a very constricted emotional world, and some people with dpdr describe feeling nothing at all, like a full automaton—the "living dead." Discussion about the precise meaning of words and the true intent of the person saying them inevitably leads down a long and winding road. Ultimately, describing dpdr symptoms is akin to describing the taste of an orange, or a peach. You can say it's tart, tangy, sweet, or comparable to something else, but no words can truly describe the taste.

As stated at the outset of this chapter, despite the limitations of words, depersonalized people have shown themselves to be quite capable of relating to each other's descriptions of symptoms, as evidenced by the burgeoning communication that has evolved in forums and chat groups on the internet. Through all venues, scientific or lay, core symptoms have long been identified, and the way of describing them usually involves intuitively understood language. To further explore the types of descriptions that clinicians are likely to draw upon during a patient assessment, let's look at the two widely used self-administered questionnaires that are very helpful in detecting and quantifying dpdr.

The Dissociative Experiences Scale

The Dissociative Experiences Scale (DES) is a 28-item questionnaire that has been very widely used over the past 35 years to detect and measure dissociative symptoms (available online). It was developed in 1986 by Drs. Eve Bernstein-Carlson and Frank Putnam, two well-known experts in the field of dissociation and trauma.[2] Each DES item is scored on a 0% to 100% scale, based on how frequently it is experienced, and the total DES score is the mean (average) of all items. In addition to its clinical usefulness, the DES has been used in thousands of research studies and has been translated into many languages. Of its 28 questions only five directly relate to dpdr experiences, and so it's quite possible for a person suffering from troubling dpdr to still score low on the total DES, which was originally designed with the more "severe" dissociative disorders like dissociative identity disorder in mind.

Still, the DES is a very helpful tool in detecting DDD: DES items indicative of dpdr are scored high, while other types of dissociative symptoms (such as amnesia or identity alteration) can be excluded if pertinent DES items are scored low. This "dissection" of dissociative symptoms is an advantage that the DES offers over questionnaires that only inquire about dpdr (see next questionnaire). An additional advantage of the DES is that it quantifies "normative" dissociation, the kind of dissociation that is present in all people to varying degrees and commonly referred to as "absorption." Absorption is the state of mind we all find ourselves in when watching a good movie, driving on a familiar highway, or daydreaming while attending a boring lecture. Yet, those with DDD manifest *higher* absorption scores compared to "healthy control" research participants, reflecting their general dissociation-proneness.[3]

The five DES items typically scored high by those with DDD are items 7, 11, 12, 13, and 28.[3] Perusing the questions readily reveals why this is:

7. Some people have the experience of feeling as though they are standing next to themselves or watching themselves do something, almost as if they were looking at another person.
11. Some people have the experience of looking in a mirror and not recognizing themselves.
12. Some people have the experience of feeling that other people, objects, and the world around them are not real.
13. Some people have the experience of feeling that their body does not seem to belong to them.
28. Some people feel as if they are looking at the world through a fog, so that people and objects appear far away or unclear.

For a clinician without extensive expertise in dissociative presentations, the DES is a valuable scale to master. Learning the questions, which are designed to be very "user-friendly," can help inquire about dissociative symptoms in a more refined manner, using language that patients can readily relate to. Another option is to administer this quick scale to patients and review their responses: formal scoring is easy enough but not even necessary—a bird's-eye view will reveal what types of dissociative experiences are present, or absent.

The Cambridge Depersonalization Scale

To better clarify the nature of DDD, psychiatrists Mauricio Sierra and German Berrios reviewed the constants and stability of older writings describing depersonalization against our contemporary take on DDD.[4] Using the year 1946 as the dividing line, the investigators examined 200 cases of depersonalization from the medical literature between 1898 and 1996 (two historical groups of approximately 100 cases per 50-year period) and compared them to a contemporary patient group recruited by the investigators. In addition to the general descriptions of unreality, specific key symptoms emerged:

- Changes in sensory experience (vision, hearing, touch, taste, smell)
- Emotional numbing
- Changes in body experience
- Changes in the subjective experience of memory
- Loss of feelings of agency
- Feelings of thought emptiness
- Inability to evoke images
- Heightened self-observation
- Distortions in the experiencing of time

By quantifying all the above symptoms within the study's three groups (two historical and one current), an intriguing conclusion was reached: "The findings reported in this paper suggest that the phenomenology of depersonalization has remained stable over the last 100 years. In spite of this, the clinical profile of published case reports has been found to vary in specific ways. These variations are likely to have been determined by changing theoretical views on depersonalization. Guided by theory, clinicians were sensitized to perceive and report the same clinical phenomena in selective ways" (p. 635). Simply put, theory-driven biases changed over time, and led to an over-emphasis of certain aspects of dpdr while neglecting others. For example, thought emptiness and difficulty evoking images figured prominently in the pre-1946 historical group, heightened self-observation in the post-1946 historical group, while emotional numbing and loss of agency were comparable across all three groups.

Informed by their historical explorations, Sierra and Berrios published in 2000 a self-administered questionnaire called the Cambridge Depersonalization Scale (CDS).[5] The 29-item CDS specifically detects and measures dpdr experiences (as opposed to any other types of dissociative experiences) and over the past 20 years has become our most thorough and reliable measure of dpdr. Each of its 29 questions is rated as the sum of its frequency (how often it occurs) and duration (how long it lasts). Total CDS score is calculated as the sum of all items. The CDS is presented in its entirety below.

Frequency	Duration
0 = never	1 = few seconds
1 = rarely	2 = few minutes
2 = often	3 = few hours
3 = very often	4 = about a day
4 = all the time	5 = more than a day
	6 = more than a week

1. Out of the blue, I feel strange, as if I were not real or as if I were cut off from the world.
2. What I see looks "flat" or "lifeless", as if I were looking at a picture.
3. Parts of my body feel as if they didn't belong to me.
4. I have found myself not being frightened at all in situations which normally I would find frightening or distressing.
5. My favorite activities are no longer enjoyable.
6. Whilst doing something I have the feeling of being a "detached observer" of myself.
7. The flavour of meals no longer gives me a feeling of pleasure or distaste.
8. My body feels very light, as if it were floating on air.

9. When I weep or laugh, I do not seem to feel any emotions at all.

10. I have the feeling of not having any thoughts at all, so that when I speak it feels as if my words were being uttered by an "automaton".

11. Familiar voices (including my own) sound remote and unreal.

12. I have the feeling that my hands or my feet have become larger or smaller.

13. My surroundings feel detached or unreal, as if there was a veil between me and the outside world.

14. It seems as if things that I have recently done had taken place a long time ago. For example anything which I have done this morning feels as if it were done weeks ago.

15. Whilst fully awake I have "visions" in which I can see myself outside, as if I were looking at my image in a mirror.

16. I feel detached from memories of things that have happened to me— as if I had not been involved in them.

17. When in a new situation, it feels as if I have been through it before.

18. Out of the blue, I find myself not feeling any affection towards my family and close friends.

19. Objects around me seem to look smaller or further away.

20. I cannot feel properly the objects that I touch with my hands for it feels as if it were not me who were touching them.

21. I do not seem able to picture things in my mind, for example, the face of a close friend or a familiar place.

22. When a part of my body hurts, I feel so detached from the pain that it feels as if it were "somebody else's" pain.

23. I have the feeling of being outside my body.

24. When I move it doesn't feel as if I were in charge of the movements, so that I feel "automatic" and mechanical as if I were a "robot".

25. The smell of things no longer gives me a feeling of pleasure or dislike.

26. I feel so detached from my thoughts that they seem to have a "life" of their own.

27. I have to touch myself to make sure that I have a body or a real existence.

28. I seem to have lost some bodily sensations (e.g. of hunger and thirst) so that when I eat or drink, it feels like an automatic routine.

29. Previously familiar places look unfamiliar, as if I had never seen them before.

Not surprisingly, the CDS total score is strongly correlated with the dpdr items score of the DES. While the maximum possible score on the CDS is 290, a score of at least 70 reliably discriminates those with DDD from others with conditions like anxiety disorders or temporal lobe epilepsy who experience lesser sprinklings of dpdr.[5] Though the comprehensiveness of the scale helps to map out the entire spectrum of dpdr symptoms, its length and "double scoring" can sometimes be prohibitive timewise. A much briefer version of the CDS was proposed in 2011, containing only two items (1 and 13, *unreality* of self and surroundings), and has been shown to quickly and reliably detect clinically significant dpdr in large community and research samples.[6]

Grouping Dpdr Symptoms

The types of experiences included in the 29 questions of the CDS deserve a closer look. First, the questionnaire includes a few queries about a variety of derealization experiences relating to a sense of unfamiliarity and estrangement from the surrounding world. These often accompany depersonalization, and at times may be the most prominent (items 2, 13, 19, 29). But the questionnaire primarily focuses on a variety of depersonalization experiences: detachment from one's body (3, 23, 27); from one's thoughts (10, 26); from one's perceptions such as vision, hearing, smell, taste, and touch (2, 11, 7, 20, 25); from internal sensations like hunger and thirst (28); from pain, a symptom known as analgesia (22); an altered sense of time (14); a difficulty evoking past memories (16, 21); and what is known as hypoemotionality or emotional numbness, a dampening of one's feelings, positive or negative, such as sadness, anger, love, and happiness (4, 5, 9, 18). Patients may experience symptoms from many or few of the above domains; some will claim to suffer from only one symptom or a limited number of symptoms—sometimes they find it hard to believe that all these experiences are encompassed under the same disorder, yet there is no evidence to the contrary.

In 2008, an analysis was published statistically "deconstructing" the CDS into its major components in a large group of 394 individuals who endorsed dpdr via an internet survey.[7] The group had an average CDS total score of 120, well above the minimum cutoff score of 70 recommended for detecting DDD; the two CDS items used for brief screening had robust average scores around 7. Five CDS domains emerged through the deconstruction:

- Numbing
- Unreality of the self
- Perceptual alterations
- Unreality of surroundings
- Temporal disintegration

These five domains distill and condense all the many dpdr experiences discussed in this chapter, and as such are clinically useful when inquiring about dpdr in a well-paced yet thorough fashion. They encompass the general domain of "unreality" of self and world, as well as feelings, sensations, and time perception. Yet nothing reveals the pain and dysfunction of DDD like the poignant quotations from patients describing their unique and disturbing subjective experiences within each of these five domains.

Unreality of Self

My thoughts are separate from my body, as if my mind exists in one place and my physicality in another. I see myself doing things, like a machine, like I'm in a movie. I go through the motions as if I'm in a play. How can I be inside myself while watching myself at the same time? Words come out of my mouth but they don't seem to be directed by me. They just come out, and sometimes I become flustered and begin to stammer or slur. My arms and legs don't feel like they're mine. How do I control them? What makes them move? I look in the mirror to try to re-center myself but I still feel like I'm in the Twilight Zone. Like a zombie, like the living dead. Am I really me? My thoughts about the depersonalization lead me on a perpetual tortured journey of questions without answers. I am always watching and analyzing everything about me, trapped in my brain. I almost "see" everything I think as if it were spelled out on a billboard. I can't stop thinking about thinking. And the more I think, the less I know. Who or what am I? Where did I come from? Where will I end up? I thought I knew once, but I feel that my answers were all illusions. I always wonder about those who kill themselves—I am already dead.

Unreality of Surroundings

Familiar things look strange and foreign. I feel like an anthropologist on another planet, studying the human species. I look at things that once meant a lot to me, and I don't understand what I saw in them that made me love them. They're just shapes, objects, things, with no personal connection to me. My old coffee mug looks no more familiar than a baby with two heads. It's all just there and it's all strange somehow. I see everything through a fog. Fluorescent lights intensify the horrible sensation and cast a deep veil over everything. I'm sealed in plastic wrap, closed off, almost deaf in the muted silence. It is as if the world were made of cellophane or glass. I feel like Alice in Wonderland. The world is inside out, upside down, and unpleasantly strange, like being trapped in a carnival fun house where mirrors distort everything.

Hypoemotionality/Numbing

I have no moods. Things that used to cause a response in me do nothing. A beautiful painting or a vivid sunset that once moved me no longer arouses me. I wanted to cry when my mother died but didn't. Not because I didn't love her, I just could not evoke how it should feel; I knew she's no longer in the world, but neither am I. I remember once feeling the change of seasons in my stomach, filled with memories and nostalgia. I can't feel all that anymore. Nothing sparks any kind of emotion in me, except possibly fear sometimes. I feel as if I am dead. I have no sense of humor but fake false smiles when necessary. I am deceiving my loved ones pretending to feel for them, to be connected and to care. My soul has been stolen from me. All I feel is a strange void. It is like a Biblical curse—my wine has turned to vinegar, food to dry tasteless powder—my soul has departed. I have died, and with this lack of feeling comes a strange unification with the cold, unfeeling night that lasts forever.

Perceptual/Sensory Alterations

I cannot feel sex. I touch my body, pinch it, rub it, to feel something. I look at my hands and wonder if they're mine; they look bigger, or smaller, or just strange. Sometimes when I'm very stressed my body gets lighter and lighter and I almost float away. It's like I leave my body entirely. Food tastes very bland, and sometimes I forget that I am thirsty. My voice sounds strange, like when I used to listen to recordings of myself. I see myself from the outside, like I'm looking at a mirror, yet when I look in the mirror it's not me that I see.

Temporal Disintegration

I have no sense of time—a thousand years can seem like an hour, a few seconds can seem like days. My memories of my past life feel like they did not happen to me. Remembering my past is like looking at photographs of someone else's life. And so I look at photographs desperately trying to evoke how I felt then, and then, and then. My most treasured memories are now so dulled—dreams feel more real than waking life. I try to evoke last night's outing, but it feels like it happened ages ago. Yet my college graduation feels like yesterday. My life as it used to be feels very far away, no longer connected to me in the string of my life. The string is cut into pieces and time warps.

4

Making the Diagnosis

Portray [people with mental illness] sympathetically, and portray them in all the richness and depth of their experience as people, not as diagnoses.

—Elyn Saks

Like any other psychiatric condition, the diagnosis of depersonalization/derealization disorder (DDD) is made clinically, by meeting with the patient and conducting a thorough evaluation. Dissociative disorders are generally known to be founded in experiences of trauma that occurred typically, but not necessarily, earlier in life (according to the latest edition of the *Diagnostic and Statistical Manual of Mental Disorders* [*DSM-5-TR*]),[1] reflecting adaptation and survival in otherwise intolerable circumstances—no matter what the price. Since the advent in 1980 of the third edition of the *Diagnostic and Statistical Manual of Mental Disorders*,[2] DDD has been classified by modern American psychiatry within the dissociative disorders. Its traumatic antecedents are more varied than those encountered in the more "severe" dissociative disorders such as dissociative identity disorder. Not only childhood maltreatment but also adulthood traumatic stressors, frightening episodes of other mental illnesses, and even drug use typically accompanied by "bad trips" can contribute to the genesis of DDD, and in some cases there may even be no apparent "cause" or trigger, at least early on (see Chapters 6 and 7).

The symptoms detailed in the previous chapter serve as the point of departure—yet to diagnose the disorder, symptoms cannot be just transient; they must be chronic. The symptoms must also not occur *only* in the context of some other condition, be it psychiatric, medical, or related to substance use (see next chapter). If, for example, depersonalization/derealization (dpdr) symptoms happen only when a person is deeply depressed, or during a period of panic attacks, or with seizures, or because a person has a brain tumor, they would not be diagnosed as having DDD. Likewise, if a person

Feeling Unreal. Second Edition. Daphne Simeon and Jeffrey Abugel, Oxford University Press. © Oxford University Press 2023. DOI: 10.1093/oso/9780197622445.003.0004

is a habitual substance user and experiences dpdr only in that context, they would still not be diagnosed with DDD.

Distress and Impairment

In addition to the presence of symptoms, a diagnosis of DDD requires that a person must experience significant distress or impairment as a result of these symptoms. Indeed, many people with DDD suffer tremendously. They typically describe that they function suboptimally, or barely at all, in school or at work, because they feel foggy, detached, blank, or obsessively preoccupied with trying to figure out their condition. They often report that their interpersonal relationships, especially the more intimate ones, are deeply perturbed because of the abnormal sense of selfhood and the distorted sense of connectedness with others. The pervasive sense of unreality and detachment may or may not be sensed by others. At times, partners or close friends may be quite aware of how cut off, flattened, or disengaged their loved one appears to be. At other times they are surprised or frustrated to hear of the condition and how it affects the patient, since everything may look fine on the surface. Still others with DDD are so socially impaired that they live in virtual seclusion.

Some people find dpdr so distressing that every living moment is a nightmare, often expressed in terms like "I have no soul," "what is the point of killing myself; I'm already dead," or "I'm not alive anymore; nothing makes a difference." Notably, these devastating feelings can be present even in the absence of depression. On the other hand, there are people with DDD, especially those who have had it as far back as they can remember or whose symptoms are more fluctuant, who are not particularly distressed and have adapted in their own ways. They describe that their dissociation is a safe and comforting place for them to retreat into, shielding them from overwhelmedness and fright. However, lower distress need not imply limited impairment; it may come with the price of social isolation or occupational difficulties.

Others may find similarities between DDD and altered states of consciousness that are actively sought out through meditation and other consciousness-altering practices (see Chapter 9), but for the typical person who finds DDD unbearably unpleasant, the sense that something about them is terribly out of kilter makes a lot more sense than any interpretations pointing toward a higher consciousness or an enlightened state. For most, these realms are something they never sought, and from which they would like to escape.

DSM-5-TR Diagnostic Criteria

According to the *DSM-5-TR*,[1] DDD is characterized by clinically significant *persistent* or *recurrent* depersonalization (experiences of unreality or detachment from one's self) and/or derealization (experiences of unreality or detachment from one's surroundings). There is no evidence of any distinction between individuals with predominantly depersonalization versus predominantly derealization symptoms. Therefore, people with DDD can have depersonalization, derealization, or both.

Persistent or recurrent episodes of *depersonalization* are characterized by "a feeling of unreality or detachment from, or unfamiliarity with, one's whole self or from aspects of the self" (Criterion A1). As discussed in the previous chapter, an individual may feel detached from their entire being ("I am no one," "I have no self"), or from aspects of the self including feelings (hypoemotionality: "I know I love my children but I don't feel it"), thoughts ("my mind is blank as if my head is filled with cotton"), the body or parts of it ("my hands doesn't feel like they're mine; I look in the mirror and I don't see me"), or internal sensations ("I never feel hunger and forget to eat"). There may also be a diminished sense of agency (feeling robotic, like an automaton, not in control of one's speech, movements, and actions). The depersonalization experience can sometimes be one of a split or divided self, with one part observing and one participating. At its most extreme form this may manifest as a full-blown "out-of-body experience," infrequently encountered in DDD.

Persistent or recurrent episodes of *derealization* are characterized by a "feeling of unreality or detachment from, or unfamiliarity with, the world, be it individuals, inanimate objects, or all surroundings" (Criterion A2). Patients may feel as they are in a fog, dream, or bubble, or as if there were a veil or glass between them and the outside world. The world around may be experienced as artificial, colorless, or lifeless. Derealization is commonly accompanied by perceptual alterations, such as visual distortions (blurriness, heightened acuity, widened or narrowed visual field, two-dimensionality or flatness, exaggerated three-dimensionality, altered distance or size of objects). Auditory distortions can also occur, whereby voices or sounds are muted or heightened, as well as alterations in taste and smell.

All these alterations of experience in DDD must be accompanied by "intact reality testing": the person knows that what they are experiencing is not, objectively, "real" (Criterion B). Additionally, there is Criterion C, which requires the presence of clinically significant distress or impairment in social, occupational, or other important areas of functioning, as discussed earlier. Finally, Criteria D and E specify other diagnoses in the presence of a diagnosis of DDD cannot be made; these are examined in the next chapter.

Other associated features characteristic of the disorder, already discussed in previous chapters, are important to note. Individuals with DDD may have difficulty describing their symptoms and may fear that they are "going crazy." Another common fear, especially but not limited to dpdr precipitated by drug use, is the fear of irreversible brain damage. A common dpdr symptom not explicitly mentioned in Criteria A and B is an altered perception of time (too fast or too slow), as well as a difficulty in vividly and emotionally recalling memories. Vague somatic complaints are quite common, such as head tightness "like a band," tingling sensations, or lightheadedness and a sense of being off-balance. Some people with DDD have intense ruminations or obsessional preoccupations with their symptoms, for example constantly thinking about whether they really exist or checking their vision to determine how things look. Varying degrees of anxiety and low mood are also common. Finally, though intentional dpdr-like experiences can be a part of meditative and ritualized practices prevalent in many religions and cultures, they do not constitute and should not be diagnosed as a clinical condition. However, when individuals who initially self-induced such states inadvertently enter a phase of uncontrolled and more chronic dpdr, as can happen on occasion, the diagnosis of DDD may be apt.

The case report that follows illustrates some of the typical features of this disorder.

The Story of Jada

Jada K., now 20, grew up as an only child with a mother who suffered from a chronic psychotic disorder. Mrs. K. was not employed, while Mr. K. was a manager at a local supermarket, working long hours and hardly ever around. Despite attempts to get Mrs. K. treatment, Jada's mother had remained largely untreated throughout the years, and never took medication on a regular basis. Jada's earliest memories were of an erratic, unpredictable, and strangely behaving mother. Mrs. K. had never been able to keep a clean and neat household. Jada recalls living in a messy, disorganized environment, with stacks of mail, clothing, and trash bags lying around everywhere. Mrs. K did not cook with any regularity, and Jada remembers having to improvise dinners from a young age, out of a mostly empty refrigerator. Despite loving Jada and never being intentionally mean or abusive toward her, Mrs. K. was unable to provide any consistent warmth, nurturing, or guidance to her daughter.

Often, Mrs. K. suffered what seemed to Jada like attacks of some sort. She would become suspicious that neighbors were plotting against her to get her out of the neighborhood. Up all night, she would lock all the windows and doors of the house, turn off the lights, and keep watch, while instructing Jada to take cover under a table or bed. The attacks could last for days, although Mrs. K.'s worse predictions never seemed to come true. Jada was terrified of both the potential danger that her mother seemed to be sensing and, as the years passed, more so of her mother's erratic behavior. She recalled numerous instances of patiently waiting for what seemed like an eternity for the crisis to pass and for her family to be able to return to some sense of normalcy. Jada had at times tried to approach her father and tell him about the happenings in the home, but he remained largely uninvolved and seemingly unable to comprehend how serious things would get. Finally, Jada gave up on him as well.

She recalls often coming home from school and having to brace herself for another evening of loneliness, pain, fear, and bewilderment. She attended the local public school, and despite her deep yearning to have relationships and fun times with her peers, she never made lasting friends. A big part of the problem, as Jada was likeable and social enough, was that Mrs. K. unwittingly hindered Jada's efforts at socialization. When Jada was invited to other students' homes, her mother would begin to worry that Jada would somehow be hurt or mistreated, and she would plead or demand that she return home. Friends sometimes asked to stop by Jada's home, but she was too ashamed to invite them over, fearing that they or their parents would catch on to her mother's bizarreness. In town, Mrs. K. had gained a reputation for being odd and people avoided her, fearing she might lash out unexpectedly, or accuse them of imaginary wrongdoings.

Jada's isolated and deprived life continued throughout elementary, middle, and high school. From those years, looking back now, she could recall a few instances of transient depersonalization. The first one occurred when she was nine or so, when her mother had her first severe paranoid crisis, locked up the house in darkness in the middle of the afternoon, and insisted that Jada hide in the basement. Jada obediently did so and remembers crouching in a corner feeling that it was all a dream. She no longer felt like the little frightened kid that she was, but like a detached observer looking at herself and emotionlessly appraising the situation. It was all unreal, she thought, happening but not really happening. The next time that she experienced depersonalization she was 13, after another of her mother's crises. Determined to do something about it, she stayed up late that night after Mrs. K. went to bed to discuss the matter with her father. When Mr. K. came home at 11 p.m. after his second shift, Jada eagerly described what her mother had been like that afternoon, trying to convince him that they should get her help at the local hospital. Her father appeared exhausted and indifferent, flatly stating, "Your mother is OK. Go to bed now." Jada again suddenly felt unreal; this could only be a dream. She remained in this state until she fell asleep very late that night, and the next morning she woke up "normal" again.

Jada experienced fleeting depersonalization for the third time when she was 16. Sarah, a friend from school, insisted on coming home with her one afternoon after class so they could work on a tough homework assignment together. Jada felt great trepidation but said nothing as they walked to her home. When they entered the house Sarah declared: "Jada, your home is a real mess!" The exclamation poignantly and painfully captured Jada's entire existence, and again she suddenly felt like all was unreal. It was as if she was no longer Jada. She felt dead, in very slowed motion, and like an automaton went through the motions of the evening long after Sarah had left. Sarah never returned; months later Jada learned through word of mouth that Sarah's parents had warned her to stay away from Mrs. K.'s house.

Jada graduated high school with average grades, little ambition, and no sense of direction or goals. She moved two hours away to live in a dorm while attending community college. The first year of college was especially tough for her. Classes were difficult, making friends was hard, and her mother often called her to warn her of unforeseen and irrational dangers. Studying amidst noise and distraction had never been a problem for Jada. But now everything, from low-volume music, to conversations in the hallways, to the sounds of the heating system, seemed to fluster and confuse her, and she was unable to concentrate. Still, she managed to find quiet corners where she could study.

Before long she started dating for the first time in her life, and by the spring she had a regular boyfriend, Ed. Ed did not treat her particularly well, and a couple months later Jada found out that he was having relationships with other young women on campus. By April, she was immensely stressed out and feared she would just not make it through the first year. Finals were approaching, her midterm grades were mediocre, Ed was aloof, and she needed to study hard in the weeks ahead. She tried to make progress, but one month before finals her father called late one night to tell her that her mother had had yet another crisis. A neighbor had called the police and Mrs. K. had ended up, involuntarily, in a hospital psychiatric service, crying, "If only Jada were here to protect me, this would never have happened."

Jada began to fade in and out of reality. She felt foggy, absent, emotionless, robotic. These experiences gradually intensified over the next few weeks. One day she went to the mall to clear her mind, only to have the crowds there seem unreal and somehow nightmarish, as if everyone was watching and judging her, even though she knew it not to be true. Inside one department store, the fluorescent lights seemed to cast a ghoulish haze on all the merchandise, and Jada became very lightheaded and momentarily exited her body and was looking down on herself standing beside a rack of summer dresses. Back at her dorm room, these experiences continued and became more frequent and intense, as if her very soul was seeping out of her body, little by little. By the end of her final exams, which she barely managed to take, Jada was in an intractable depersonalized state.

Cognizant of her movements, watching herself as if she were in a movie with the sound turned down, she packed her things and left school to go home for the summer. She walked into her old home, visited her mother who was still in the hospital, and talked with her father to find out the details of what was going on. But *she* was no longer there, for good. Alive but dead, she felt, and remained in this state all summer though her mother was soon discharged on a medication regimen and was more stable over that summer. In the fall, Jada returned to college and decided to seek help at the mental health clinic. There was still the remnant of an attitude— a determination to tackle her problems, and not let what happened to her mother happen to her too.

What is Jada's diagnosis? Selected as a straightforward case (we will be discussing more complicated cases in the next chapter), Jada is experiencing new-onset DDD. After three short-lived episodes of dpdr in her preteen and teen years, she had now become chronically depersonalized for the past five months. This is a common pattern. Jada's brief dpdr episodes had occurred at peak at times of intolerable fear and helplessness, triggered by severe crises at home. Then, in her late adolescence, she experienced the new and severe, for her, stressor of transitioning out of home to college—with its educational, social, and romantic demands that she felt she could not meet, coupled with a lot of guilt over abandoning her sick mother. This major life transition was the final straw that precipitated the prolonged dpdr episode, which met *DSM-5-TR* criteria for DDD.

Although chronically traumatized, Jada had never been particularly depressed or anxious, and had never experienced panic attacks. Though she worried about one day becoming "crazy" like her mother, there was no evidence that Jada was on a path to a psychotic disorder. She was not odd as a child and, though she only had friendly acquaintances growing up, she had always longed for deeper friendships yet her extenuating circumstances precluded them. Jada did feel unreal, but she in no way believed that she was turning into a machine or that her life was literally a dream; this is just how it all started to *feel*. When reality became too terrifying and painful, unreality somehow became a refuge. It was quite clear to her that her state was not "normal," and she opted to seek help for it.

Her fear that she might be getting ill like her mother is a common one, as the clinician she saw reassured her. Children often worry that they might somehow have "inherited" the worst of their parents and can find evidence that this might be so. The therapist also validated for Jada that she had a very adverse upbringing, continuously and relentlessly so. Both her parents, each in their own way, had failed to provide for her fundamental emotional needs and longings. In the words of Jada's newly found therapist, every child needs to feel safe, recognized, nurtured, guided, and socialized in basic and important ways—for Jada, these went unmet.

The Clinical Evaluation

As with any psychiatric or medical condition, a thorough evaluation and accurate diagnosis is crucial to a patient's understanding of what is ailing them, and for the formulation of the initial treatment plan. In the first consultation, the mental health professional may or may not know or suspect that the person coming for help is experiencing dissociation, or dpdr. This of course will depend on the nature of the referral, as well as a patient's presenting complaint, referred to in psychiatry as the "chief" complaint. Regardless, clinicians do a complete "review of systems" (another medical term), and inquire methodically about all the possible psychiatric symptoms, current and lifetime, that a person may be experiencing. In fact, no clinician will neglect to inquire about history of anxiety, depression, psychosis, substance use, suicidality, and the like. Yet, non-specialist clinicians at times fail to ask patients about dissociative symptoms, if these do not spontaneously come up—and, even worse, sometimes may not pick up on them or misconstrue them even when they do come up.

Such an omission is unfortunate and can be easily avoided by a single screening question for dissociative symptoms, as routinely asked for other kinds of psychiatric symptoms. For example, the single question *"Have you ever felt unreal or detached from yourself or your surroundings, have unusual or unaccountable gaps in your memory, or have somehow felt that that there is more than one of you?"* encompasses dpdr, amnesia, and identity alteration, and serves as an inroad to the exploration of dissociative symptoms. If a positive response is elicited for any portion of this tripartite question, further inquiry is needed. A clinician might first encourage a patient to elaborate in their own words, then ask more directed and probing questions. Some clinicians choose to administer questionnaires that tap into dissociation as part of their initial assessment, such as the Dissociative Experiences Scale (DES)[3] or the Cambridge Depersonalization Scale (CDS)[4] (see previous chapter). These scales can be very useful both in helping patients feel understood and in narrowing the diagnosis.

If a new patient is experiencing unreality or detachment, the detailed symptoms and their history are inquired about in chronological sequence. It is very important to know whether there had been episodes of dpdr before the more recent and presenting episode. Though these may or may not have been distressing enough for the patient to seek help, they are revealing for several reasons. First, they support the notion that an individual has a dissociative diathesis dating further back in time, even before manifesting clinically problematic symptoms. This helps support and strengthen the current diagnosis. Second, they facilitate the differential diagnosis (see next chapter)—if a patient had earlier, albeit more transient dpdr, the later occurrence of significant dpdr symptoms is less likely to be occurring exclusively as a part of another psychiatric disorder (this, of course, still has to be assessed). Third, while earlier and fleeting dpdr experiences may involve some detective work, they provide important clues as to the historical origins and the meanings of the dissociation.

The following example is a commonly encountered one. A 21-year-old presented with new-onset DDD over the past 10 months. Careful history-taking determined that early experiences of floating in midair had started at age 10, lasting about 15 minutes; these had occurred about a dozen times over the next few years. Further exploration revealed that this young woman had been fondled by a visiting relative the summer before fourth grade. It is reasonable to assume that this sexual transgression triggered the onset of dissociative experiences, even if these did not become more pronounced until the now young woman had to contend with deepening sexual intimacy in her first longstanding romantic relationship. In this way, the past and the present, and the links that bridge them, begin to create a meaningful, cohesive narrative.

The mental health professional will also take a detailed history of all past clinically significant dpdr episodes—the ones that lasted longer and caused distress or impairment. Just as with depression, for example, these episodes need to be mapped out with a time stamp, duration, type of onset and resolution, other concurrent psychiatric symptoms, and any precipitants or triggers for each episode that a patient can recall. This mapping of dpdr episodes alongside other conditions is crucial to diagnosis, as the next chapter will describe in detail. If it becomes clear, for example, that every dpdr episode occurred within the onset of a clinical depression, and completely lifted with its resolution or shortly thereafter, the diagnosis would be depression, and the dissociative symptoms would be a part of that clinical diagnosis. On the other hand, if only one dpdr episode occurred within the context of a depression but others did not, a different diagnosis would be warranted.

The mapping of dpdr episodes also allows the clinician to assess the greater course of the condition over time. If there has been more than one episode in a person's life so far, are the episodes becoming more or less frequent, lasting, intense, distressing and impairing, or even more "autonomous," in the sense that over time they are less dependent on identifiable triggers? These are important considerations because they hint at prognosis—how a patient is likely to fare in the future (treatment considerations aside). A worsening progression with time is generally more concerning, and may affect the treatment plan. It is also helpful to find out if the predominant dpdr symptoms have changed in any notable way over time. Sometimes this is not the case, but other times it is. For example, a patient who initially experienced only derealization might, over time, become increasingly depersonalized. Though this evolution may not impact the diagnosis or treatment plan per se, it is important to discuss with the patient who is worried about the meanings of this development, or who finds the present symptoms more, or less, distressing than earlier ones.

It is also useful to elicit further aspects of the dpdr episodes—exacerbating and alleviating factors, as well as fluctuations in daily intensity. Most patients can list several factors, internal or external ones, that worsen or lighten up their dpdr experiences. They display commonalities across individuals but may also differ in unique ways. For example, for some sunlight or bright lights worsen symptoms, whereas for others dusk and nighttime do so. Or for some being with other people consistently helps, while others predictably feel worse. Knowing what makes symptoms better or worse can help shape treatment strategies (see Chapter 12). As importantly, all these factors begin to paint a psychological picture of what the dissociation is really about, on the path to deeper psychotherapeutic exploration.

Though not an exhaustive list, some common clinical, emotional, inter-personal, and physical exacerbating factors are as follows. Any coexisting psychiatric symptoms can worsen dpdr: anxiety, panic attacks, depression, obsessive-compulsive disorder (OCD) attacks, even episodes of bipolar highs or lows. Emotionally, stress tends to be a common trigger, though individuals may be vulnerable to different types of stressors; what is highly stressful to one person may not be so for another. Disturbing and over-whelming emotional states can also be triggering, including negative emo-tional states of sadness, loneliness, fear, shame, and despair, to name just a few. Paradoxically, positive emotional states can be triggering for some patients as well. These may include feelings of closeness, happiness, excite-ment, hopefulness, or other wellbeing, particularly when there is a psycho-logical history rendering such good feelings unsafe.

Interpersonally, the presence of close or casual others, when underlying conflicts and dangers are present, can be triggering, as can be the absence of others and the sense of aloneness. Understandably, DDD can be extremely isolating at times. The "others" in one's life—who they are and how they fit in—often play a big role that needs to be understood. They may be family, ro-mantic partners, sexual encounters, co-workers, bosses, and so on.

Physical factors often cited as worsening dpdr include poor sleep, lighting conditions (brighter, dimmer, or artificial such as fluorescent lights), time of day, quality of sleep, exertion, and states of tension or relaxation. Alleviating factors also need to be investigated and understood; understandably, some are the reverse of the exacerbating factors.

Dpdr symptom intensity is also very important for the clinician to assess—for example, whether symptoms fluctuate over the course of the day, or over weeks, or whether they are like a flat line of sorts; and whether this pattern has changed over the years. This matters to patients, naturally. Most find it more distressing when there is little or no respite from the intensity of symptoms. It also matters prognostically and treatment-wise. In general, though no generalizations are absolute, individuals with more longstanding and constant-intensity DDD can be harder to treat. There are a couple likely reasons for this. First, it is an indicator of chronicity, and any psychiatric condition that has been present for a longer time can take longer to treat. Second, a clinician generally has less to "work with," both outside the sessions and within them, when a person's symptoms do not fluctuate (see psychotherapy chapters).

By the end of the initial evaluation, the mental health professional will be able to offer feedback regarding the diagnosis, or diagnoses; discuss the relationship between the various diagnoses; present a summary of DDD's chronology, course, and prognosis; and propose a treatment plan. More tentative first impressions are shared as such and are subject to further exploration and clarification. And treatment is about to get off the ground.

5

Differential Diagnosis

Bedside manners are no substitute for the right diagnosis.
—Alfred P. Sloan

For an individual to be diagnosed with depersonalization/derealization disorder (DDD), depersonalization/derealization (dpdr) experiences need to be persistent or recurrent; reality testing must be intact; and the symptoms must cause significant distress or impairment (Criteria A, B, and C in the latest edition of the *Diagnostic and Statistical Manual of Mental Disorders* [*DSM-5-TR*]).[1] Also, the symptoms must not be attributable to ongoing substance use or to a medical condition (Criterion D). The differential diagnosis of DDD involves assessing whether other psychiatric disorders are present in the patient at the time of the dpdr episodes and, if so, determining whether these other disorders might better account for the dpdr symptoms. In such a case, a diagnosis of DDD would not be made (Criterion E).

Symptoms of anxiety, panic, and depression can sometimes mimic dpdr, or be frank dpdr. For example, in deeply depressed people feelings of numbness, deadness, or apathy are common, and can be trickier to distinguish from dpdr than more straightforward feelings of sadness, hopelessness, or despair. Symptoms of dizziness and lightheadedness are common in severe anxiety or panic but may also be associated with dpdr. Further complicating matters, dpdr comprises one of the 13 symptoms of panic attacks, more likely to be present if the panic attacks are severe. Some people with dpdr become obsessively preoccupied with their unreality experiences and even develop rituals for "checking" the presence or the changing intensity of their symptoms, moment to moment. In all these situations, a non-specialist clinician who is more familiar with depression, anxiety, and obsessions and compulsions may unwittingly be biased to detect the latter and not take notice of dpdr.

Feeling Unreal. Second Edition. Daphne Simeon and Jeffrey Abugel, Oxford University Press. © Oxford University Press 2023. DOI: 10.1093/oso/9780197622445.003.0005

Major psychiatric disorders that need to be differentiated from DDD include the anxiety disorders, major depressive disorder (MDD), obsessive-compulsive disorder (OCD), posttraumatic stress disorder (PTSD), psychotic disorders, and other dissociative disorders. Even if a doctor establishes that a patient does have clinical dpdr episodes, another one of these disorders may be present and at play: DDD can *only* be diagnosed if dpdr experiences clearly preceded the onset of the other disorder, or remain present after it resolves. As such, DDD cannot be diagnosed when dpdr occurs *only* during panic attacks; in this scenario the diagnosis would be one of panic disorder. On the other hand, it is not uncommon for dpdr to first occur in the context of new-onset panic attacks, or as panic disorder progresses and worsens. A diagnosis of DDD is then made if dpdr is pronounced and extends well beyond the actual panic attacks, or persists after the panic disorder has remitted or been successfully treated.

Dpdr may also occur during episodes of clinical (major) depression; a diagnosis of DDD would be made only if the dpdr episode clearly began before the depression, or continued well after the depression remitted. When it comes to OCD, the obsessional thinking and compulsive checking encountered in some with DDD do *not* constitute OCD. There needs to be evidence of other typical obsessive-compulsive symptoms like washing, cleaning, counting, checking, arranging, and the like—*unrelated* to dpdr themes.

Dpdr may be present in people who suffer from PTSD. In recognition of this long-known occurrence, the *DSM-5* was the first edition of the manual to demarcate a particular "subtype" of PTSD, the dissociative subtype, characterized by prominent dpdr in addition to the more classic PTSD symptoms. Dpdr, in this context, merits a diagnosis of PTSD rather than DDD.

The clinician also determines whether dpdr is accompanied by other dissociative experiences, such as amnesia or identity alteration (see Dissociative Experiences Scale, Chapter 3).[2] If other pathological dissociation symptoms are present, the diagnosis will be a dissociative disorder other than DDD, such as dissociative amnesia or dissociative identity disorder.

The presence of intact reality testing is essential for differentiating DDD from any psychotic disorder. Positive-symptom schizophrenia occasionally poses a diagnostic challenge vis-à-vis DDD, for example when nihilistic delusions are present. If a person states that they are dead or that the world does not exist, this could be either a subjective "as if" experience that the individual does not truly believe, or it could be a conviction; this crucial distinction must be established. Similarly, negative symptoms of schizophrenia (the "5 As" of affective flattening, alogia, anhedonia, asociality, and avolition) can be the only schizophrenia symptoms present in the early phase of the illness, and may mimic dpdr—patients need to be carefully assessed for any suspicion of prodromal psychosis before a DDD diagnosis is made.

Finally, mental disorders may in fact be due to an underlying medical condition or to ongoing substance use (Criterion D); this possibility should never be overlooked. DDD is not diagnosed if dpdr is associated *only* with substance intoxication or withdrawal. If dpdr experiences do not "clear" outside of the substance use, once intoxication or withdrawal is no longer at play, the situation is more suspect of DDD. At the same time, it is not uncommon for a clinical dpdr episode to be precipitated by a drug ingestion, even an isolated one[3] (see next chapter). A DDD diagnosis is usually easy to establish in this scenario, because individuals with drug-triggered dpdr almost always become intensely phobic and aversive to the offending substance and actively avoid it.

For any person presenting with dpdr, features such as onset after age 40, the presence of atypical symptoms, or an atypical course can be suggestive of an underlying medical condition. In such cases, it is essential to perform a thorough medical and neurological evaluation, which may include standard laboratory studies, various viral titers, an electroencephalogram (EEG), vestibular testing, visual testing, sleep studies, and brain imaging. Some of the more common medical problems that can manifest with dpdr are concussions; seizures; brain tumors; Lyme disease and other post-viral syndromes, including COVID-19;[4] and sleep apnea. If the suspicion of an underlying seizure disorder proves difficult to confirm with a simple EEG, an extended EEG recording may be indicated; though temporal lobe epilepsy is most commonly implicated, parietal and frontal lobe epilepsy may also be culprits.[5]

The following three patient cases bring to life some key points in the differential diagnosis of DDD.

The Story of Samesh

Samesh was 15 when he experienced his first episode of depression. Up to then he had been a happy and well-adjusted child. Those who knew him described him as introspective, thoughtful, deep, and mature beyond his years. By high school, Samesh was an avid reader who loved to ponder the complexities of relationships, the "human condition," life, death, and the question of an afterworld. At moments in his teenage years he had felt overwhelmed by thoughts of the vastness of the universe, the endlessness of time, and the minuteness of individual human presence. He wrote poignant essays in English classes, which he sometimes read out loud in class or in school competitions. He was in no sense pathologically troubled, however. He loved to have a good time, had several truly close friends, enjoyed tennis, and followed current events more closely than most boys his age.

His mother was a warm and reflective woman, who despite her interest in and earlier career teaching English literature, decided to devote her time to raising her children: Samesh and his younger brother by two years, Aarush. She was an involved and sensitive mother, whom both children felt comfortable approaching to talk about their hurts and worries. Samesh's father was a successful businessman, who worked long hours but was at home often enough to be a good dad, always conveying deep affection for his children. The parents' marriage had, at moments, felt tense to Samesh, but for the most part it was loving and harmonious.

Then, seemingly out of nowhere, the depression struck. In the winter of ninth grade, Samesh felt a proverbial black cloud begin to enshroud him. He lost all interest in school, tennis, and his friends, and his usual pondering of the nature of existence took on a heavy, morbid weight. Like people of all ages, Samesh had known brief moments of sadness, or discouragement, or self-doubt. But they had been fleeting, and usually tied to a specific event. This was different. "It was so much beyond anything I had ever felt that it was impossible to explain," he recalls. "It was like my ability to *feel* anything at all hopeful or positive had been taken away. Things I had loved and enjoyed were now meaningless and it took too much energy to even think about them."

As the condition progressed, Samesh lost his appetite and a considerable amount of weight over the next few months. Sleeping with any kind of regularity became impossible. Often, he would awaken with a start hours before the alarm was set to go off. He lay awake with eyes wide open, worrying about his illness and the nature of his own place in the universe, until the alarm finally rang. Then he would want to shut it off and sleep for the rest of the day. He continued going to school, though he wanted to just stay in bed hiding all day. His interest in his classes waned, and his homework was sloppy and hastily completed. Consequently, his grades began to drop.

Even more disturbing, his mind questioned who and what he was with relentless rumination. He felt unreal, like an actor in a play, going through the motions of daily life without any sense that he was an active participant in charge of his thoughts and feelings. Today, he vividly recalls sitting in English literature class, which he normally loved, and watching the whole scene like a spectator, totally removed. "I began to wonder if this was what it was like to be dead. Although I was certain that whatever death held, it had to be better than this."

"Ironically," Samesh adds, "in English class we were going over Hamlet's 'To Be or Not to Be' soliloquy. But I now saw it through changed eyes, because while I'd heard those lines a zillion times, like everyone else, now I really knew what Hamlet was saying."

This identification with a torn and troubled Hamlet brought little consolation at the time, however. By February, Samesh was profoundly depressed and he wanted his life to be over. He dreaded the thought of the lifetime full of work and relationships that lay ahead. He wished he were an old man, near death, with nothing to look forward to but the bliss of eternal night. But even then, as Hamlet observed, within endless sleep lay the possibility of dreams, or nightmares. "I was frozen in fear of life, and just as afraid of death," Samesh recalls. "All I could do was try to feel normal, act normal, and pray that one day I would *be* normal."

Despite his attempts to conceal these thoughts from his parents, it was clear to them that something was dreadfully wrong. Ultimately swayed by his mother's persistence, Samesh finally confided in her. He told her that he no longer felt like a person, but rather like some kind of "robot-like thing," painfully operating through each day while awaiting its end. Samesh's parents were rightfully alarmed and took him to see the school counselor. The counselor concluded that Samesh was deeply depressed but could not pinpoint any obvious trigger or reason. Samesh's mother revealed that her own mother had a serious history of what must have been depressions, not diagnosed as such in those days, only to end up chronically institutionalized, and ultimately dying in a mental hospital. Neither Samesh's parents nor his brother had ever suffered from depressive episodes.

Samesh began meeting with the counselor weekly, discussing how he felt and how he could strengthen his coping skills to make it through. The counselor explained to him the cold facts about clinical depression, including statistics inferring that it would lift in time on its own. But he did not pick up on Samesh's specific depersonalization symptoms. By late March, indeed

Samesh's mood began to improve, and by May, he no longer felt completely incapable of feeling good. "Somehow, the utter hopelessness began to lift. I started little by little to regain a sense of pleasure over little things and big things too," he recalls. His concentration improved, as did his homework, and his grades picked up for his finals. He started going out with his friends again, his energy and appetite came back, and he began to look forward again to each day with hope of steady improvement.

Samesh was still not completely himself, however. His own, private voice in his head seemed somehow louder, and somehow separate from his body. He continued to feel as if he were going through each day like a robot, watching himself as if from outside of his body, wondering who he really was. Before, he *knew* who he was. Now, inexplicably, the knowledge that he was an individual person was there, but not a clear *feeling* of "Me." Samesh attempted to describe these funny feelings to his counselor in terms of *The Twilight Zone*: "I told him about an episode where a little girl fell through a wall into another dimension. I explained that I felt like I had fallen into another dimension but hadn't come completely back out. I felt like most of me was back in the real world, but part of me was stuck on the other side, watching."

The counselor reassured him that this was just his depression getting better, and no longer met with him after school was dismissed in June. During that summer, Samesh continued to feel horrendously detached, even though he was no longer depressed. He gave up trying to describe this feeling to his family, as they only reassured him, with the best intentions, that he was on the path to recovery. By the fall and the start of the next school year, Samesh started to feel more real again. He recalls walking to school one morning in October and distinctly feeling, in the crisp autumn air looking at the first yellowing leaves, that he was himself—the Samesh he knew. It was as if his spirit has decided to re-enter his body once again. From that day on, he felt "normal," free of psychological problems for the next few years. He did not forget it all, but he was able to put his dark time behind him, graduate high school, and leave home excitedly for a prestigious college town.

From the outset, he loved college and did well. He was popular, and before long had a girlfriend. Life was good for a while. Then, halfway into his sophomore year, depression again began to resurface. The symptoms were just like the first time, and again, there was no apparent cause. Depersonalization accompanied the depression. Like a pair of thieves, Samesh's worst enemies had returned together, attempting to steal his soul once more. But this time Samesh saw them coming. He sought help at the university's mental health service right away. He was diagnosed with clinical depression by the psychiatrist on staff. Medication was recommended to expedite his recovery, given his overall good adaptation, absence of major triggers, and serious family history of depression evidenced in his grandmother.

After about four weeks on antidepressant medication, Samesh began to feel better, and within another month he was back to his usual non-depressed self. The cloud of despair lifted, he slept and woke up without much difficulty, and he felt hopeful about the future. However, the depersonalization remained as strong as ever. He continued not to feel solidly grounded in himself; he was Samesh but he wasn't. His head felt hollow, as if it were full of air. Thoughts running through his brain again seemed somehow foreign and overly present, even though there was no real deviation in their content. Thinking just *felt* different, as if coming from somewhere else. And if they weren't coming from Samesh, where were they coming from?

Praying for the day when this last unsettling disturbance would lift away as the depression had, he resumed a robot-like existence of going through the motions of his college life, getting up, going to classes, working out, meeting friends, and trying to show love and affection toward his girlfriend. When he described how he felt to his psychiatrist, his family, and his girlfriend, they all suggested that he might still be depressed. But he knew that the depression was one thing, and this was another. And there was no way to relay the difference to them.

The intensity of his depersonalization was relentless. In vain, he tried to describe how he no longer felt like a live person, but one of the "walking dead." Ultimately, realizing the pain it caused others to hear this, and the pain it caused him to not feel understood, Samesh gave up on reaching out. Still on his antidepressant, he continued feeling depersonalized for the next year. When Samesh came home for the summer, his parents recommended he see another psychiatrist. This doctor felt that Samesh's depression might not be receiving adequate treatment, so he "boosted" his antidepressant regimen—to no avail. Samesh continued to feel as depersonalized as ever. By August, he was losing hope, wondering if he would live like this for the rest of his life.

Then one night, he surfed the internet looking for whatever he could find relating to experiences of unreality and stumbled upon the term "depersonalization." Despite his numbness to everything lately, his eyes watered as he realized that he was, for the first time ever, encountering others like himself, depersonalized people suffering from a condition that most knew nothing about. He read everything he could about depersonalization and realized at last that he wasn't going insane. nor did he have some brain quirk that no one else in the world had ever had. He returned to school in the fall, his symptoms unchanged, but a little more optimistic to know what was ailing him. He shared his research with his parents and girlfriend, who also felt very relieved to better understand what Samesh had been talking about for so long and began to do their own research on the condition and look for a doctor to treat him.

Samesh carries two diagnoses, MDD and DDD, according to the *DSM-5-TR*.[1] He has had two episodes of serious clinical depression; the first one resolved spontaneously and the second one with antidepressant medication. But Samesh also suffers from DDD: he felt depersonalized *not only* during the periods when he was depressed, but rather his depersonalization lasted for months the first time, and for over a year the second time, after his depression had clearly remitted. People can feel dissociated when they are depressed (indeed, dpdr is the last item on the 21-item Hamilton Depression Rating Scale), but as the depression clears, the dissociation typically does so as well. In such cases, an additional diagnosis of DDD is not called for. According to the *DSM*, the diagnosis of DDD can be made only when the symptoms have clearly been present outside of an occurrence of another disorder such as depression.

No previously unknown triggers were later uncovered in Samesh's case. Some people can become clinically depressed without any apparent precipitating stressor. This is more common if there is a family history of depression, like Samesh's severely depressed grandmother. And what about a trigger for his depersonalization? In Samesh's mind the depersonalization was fueled by the depression itself. The depth of his despair and his incapacity to make any sense of what was going on internally, despite his deeply introspective nature, or maybe even fueled by it, left him feeling like he no longer knew himself. The endless ruminations about his own existence when he was deeply depressed might also have fueled or emboldened his dissociated state. He felt profoundly estranged from the self he had always known, a stranger trapped in his old body and mind that were now experiencing inexplicable thoughts, feelings, and physical symptoms beyond his comprehension. As he later explained to his doctor, he believed that the darkness and despair of depression was the trauma that triggered his depersonalization.

Many people with DDD tell stories similar to Samesh's. For years, case reports have appeared in the psychiatric literature of people who started out with a straightforward episode of depression that then left them chronically depersonalized after the depression resolved. One large series of patients with DDD reported that in about one-fifth of all DDD cases,[3] dpdr symptoms were initially triggered by a severe episode of another mental illness, one that presumably both induced deep fear and greatly perturbed the sense of self-hood and identity. A very similar scenario to Samesh's story with depression and DDD can unfold with disorders other than depression, such as panic disorder or OCD.

The Story of Evan

When he was 29 years old, Evan visited a psychiatrist for the first time. It was also the first time in his life that he was involved in a serious relationship with a woman. Holly, his girlfriend for about a year, had come to realize that Evan suffered when they were sexually intimate. In the beginning, her impressions were vague and unformed. Somehow, Evan seemed suddenly detached and uninvolved when in the midst of a sexual encounter. He lost his usual affection, acted distant and mechanical, and seemed almost relieved when it was all over. Later, or the next day, he seemed to revert to his usual self.

After a few months, Holly began to trust her impressions more. And because she also felt more comfortable with Evan, she decided to talk to him about her experience. She told him what she thought and felt, and to her surprise he readily, and with some relief, acknowledged that something very unusual always happened when they were intimate, and also at other times that she had not been aware of. Evan revealed that when they were intimate sexually, he would suddenly feel unreal and detached, as if he were leaving his body and observing the scene as a third party. He almost felt like he was floating over their bed, watching all that was transpiring without any emotional involvement. He knew very well that he was still himself, but his actions became perfunctory and he merely went through the motions of intimacy without any sense of involvement or participation. Although very used to this scenario, he knew it wasn't normal. But it was all he had ever known since he first became sexually active at 17. Now it distressed him greatly because he wanted to feel, and because he really cared for Holly. The detachment would typically stay with him until well after their encounters ended, often until he woke up the next morning, and sometimes for a few days after.

Sexual intimacy was not the only circumstance that made Evan feel detached, he confided to Holly. For many years, he had suffered episodes of dpdr lasting from minutes to days in settings where he somehow felt threatened, closed in, or violated. He felt very guilty that being intimate with his loved one seemed to be such a circumstance. He described an incident that occurred about a year earlier when his boss had become very angry and out of line with him. Evan was a competent and well-respected computer programmer, steadily employed with a large software company for the past four years. Once his boss, whose behavior was unpredictable and erratic, became enraged at Evan because he had failed to promptly address a major software problem being experienced by an important client. He lashed out at Evan, screaming "I know what you are all about. You have it coming." Evan suddenly felt out of this world, leaving the scene as it were and watching like a detached observer. He felt nothing, was too frozen to respond, and walked around like a zombie for a few days until the situation was cleared and his boss apologized for his coarse behavior. "Other people I know would have lashed back, or at least taken the issue to a higher-up. But I just disappeared inside. I went into a state of nothingness, no mood at all, as if I were dead," Evan recalls.

Holly asked Evan if he had any idea what these experiences might be all about. She had heard of nothing like them before and was frightened, although she did her best to be understanding and supportive. Evan agreed that his experiences were weird, and that he had never heard of anyone complaining of such states. This caused him even more worry. With Holly's prompting and persistence, Evan agreed to see a psychiatrist. Reluctantly, he made an appointment with Dr. Krast, who had been highly recommended to him by a good friend. Evan went to his first appointment, frightened but determined to get help. He described to Dr. Krast all that he had told Holly. The doctor listened attentively, encouraging Evan to go on whenever he stopped himself to reflect on the seeming absurdity of his experiences.

The doctor then told Evan that there was a name for the condition he was describing—"depersonalization." Evan had never heard of the term, and was relieved, almost joyous for a moment, to feel that not only was he not crazy or unique, but that his condition was known enough for this doctor to recognize his symptoms and give them a name. "Depersonalization?" he wondered. It seemed a very befitting term for just what he felt: like he was not a person, his own person, every time "this state" came upon him. Dr. Krast asked Evan when it had all started. Evan could not quite say, because he had had these experiences fleetingly as far back as he could remember, even before starting grade school. As distressing as the condition was for him, it was terribly familiar to him: something he had lived with all his life. Dr. Krast then asked about his early life and memories.

Evan had been an only child, who had never known his father (the father had abandoned his mother when Evan was three months old, and never saw either of them again). Evan remembered growing up very isolated, alone with his mother whose own parents lived far away. In his early years he had had little contact with any other adults or children. Dr. Krast then probed further into Evan's childhood. With great shame, but little trouble remembering, Evan revealed that his mother sometimes did "strange" things to him. Every night when she gave him a bath, she would caress him all over in ways that made him feel very uneasy. She called him endearing names, which he recalled with a bitter taste—they were too much, though he knew she loved him, and she had never been "bad" or violent. A couple times his mother even told Evan, when he misbehaved, that he "had it coming" before engaging in the usual bathing ritual. By the time Evan was eight or so, his mother's ritual gradually diminished and ended. He had never told anyone, and even though he recalled them vividly with a secret sense of shame, he had never given them much thought. He was not even sure how common or not such happenings were.

Dr. Krast revealed to Evan that they were, in fact, unusual and could well account for his lifelong depersonalization symptoms. He explained that for some people, becoming detached from intolerable experiences and feeling as if they were not really partaking in them was a way of adapting to very disturbing circumstances beyond their control. Dr. Krast explained it was not surprising that situations in Evan's life reminiscent of unwanted and threatening intimate interactions still triggered depersonalization. This included his current relationship with Holly. The doctor recommended that Evan continue to see him for talk therapy, in order to help him better understand and work through his early trauma and the symptoms it had left him with.

Evan suffers from DDD. He has experienced many bouts of classic depersonalization symptoms for his entire life. His episodes have varied in duration over the years, from fleeting when he was little to short-lived as he grew older, and were predictably triggered by reminders of feeling closed in, degraded, or sexually exposed. His last episode, since meeting Holly, has been the most persistent one to date; it was clinically significant because it was very distressing and impaired his capacity for genuine intimacy. Furthermore, Evan has intact reality testing about his depersonalization: he knows he is still himself and that his unusual perceptions are just subjective experiences that are not "real" other than for his inner world. Outside of the triggered episodes, Evan does not have odd perceptual experiences, and is quite social. There is thus no evidence that he might be experiencing a prodromal psychotic disorder.

Might Evan be suffering from another psychiatric disorder related to his traumatic history? He certainly could be, which is why Dr. Krast took an exhaustive history to delineate the full nature and extent of Evan's symptoms. For example, given the early sexual trauma, Evan could be experiencing other dissociative symptoms in addition to depersonalization. The doctor asked Evan if he ever "lost time"—that is, could not account for time periods of minutes to hours—or if he ever had "fugues," episodes where he found himself at a different place without knowing why or how he got there. People with dissociative amnesia experience such symptoms: when they "come to" after an episode, they have no idea how the time elapsed and what they were doing during it. Evan denied this; although during his deepest depersonalized moments he could be "checked out," with a blank mind, he always has some basic awareness of time and its passing.

Dr. Krast also asked him about identity shifts. People who have suffered early childhood abuse sometimes experience themselves in profoundly different ways at different moments, almost as if they are different people. At its extreme, these distinct states may have different names, appearances, ages, feelings, behaviors, and memories, and are known as dissociated self-states or identities. If a person does not have amnesia for these different alter states, they are diagnosed as suffering from "other specified dissociative disorder" in the *DSM-5-TR*. If, in its more extreme form, a person has no memory for at least some of these alter states, then the diagnosis is *DSM-5-TR* dissociative identity disorder (known to some by its old name, multiple personality disorder). Evan denied such altered states—no matter how depersonalized, he always feels he is himself, but a very unreal and deadened self. Evan then did not appear to suffer from another dissociative disorder. To be more certain, Dr. Krast also administered the Dissociative Experiences Scale, and Evan scored high only on items related to dpdr.[2]

What about PTSD? PTSD has become well known to the lay public in recent times, with the growing awareness of the detrimental impact of major traumatic events like assault, rape, combat, and war on mental wellbeing. PTSD became a part of everyone's awareness after the terrorist attack on the World Trade Center in September 2001, and a lot has been written about posttraumatic symptoms in the aftermath. For a person to suffer from PTSD, they must have "re-experiencing" intrusion symptoms (bad memories, nightmares, flashbacks); avoidance of anything or anyone reminding them of the trauma; persistent negative cognitions about the self; and hyperarousal symptoms (trouble sleeping, excessive vigilance, and startle). PTSD can result from childhood maltreatment as well, especially if the trauma was horrific enough to threaten basic safety and survival. Evan denied PTSD symptoms for the most part, except for some intrusive memories when having sex, and a certain "watchfulness" in relationships. He did not have PTSD, Dr. Krast concluded with confidence. If Evan had met diagnostic criteria for PTSD, then he would be diagnosed with PTSD "dissociative subtype" as per the *DSM-5-TR*, given his prominent dpdr symptoms.

Could Evan be just anxious or depressed? Countless people suffering from primary depersonalization are told, when they finally decide to seek help, that they are *simply* "anxious" or "depressed." Evan was fortunate in that Dr. Krast was quite familiar with his condition. Someone who is experiencing anxiety and depression should be able to admit to these, if not spontaneously, at least when asked the right kinds of questions by a professional. A person who has considerable anxiety will acknowledge feeling nervous, irritable, worrying a lot, feeling tired, on edge, or wired when trying to fall asleep, and may even describe physical symptoms like shakiness, shortness of breath, or frequent urination. Someone who is depressed, like Samesh, can usually acknowledge low mood and changes in sleep, appetite, energy level, concentration, and pleasure in day-to-day activities. Evan denied any pronounced symptoms of depression or anxiety. Though he admitted to feeling down or anxious at times, these symptoms were not intense or lasting enough to warrant a psychiatric diagnosis, and directly related to the dpdr and the struggles within the relationship with Holly.

The Story of Fen

Fen was a 21-year-old college junior majoring in fine arts at a large state university. She was bright, attractive, ambitious, and sociable, and described her upbringing as uneventful. She was the second of four children raised in a small midwestern town, and her parents were still happily married. She got along well with both parents and was particularly close to her sister Jane, who was two years younger. Fen did well in school, was athletic, and had many friends. She had never felt particularly troubled, other than the ups and downs of normal teenagers.

Prior to a fateful day that was to come, she had tried marijuana twice in her life. The first time she was in tenth grade, when she and her friends were at a party one Saturday and she took a few "tokes" of a friend's joint. She did not feel much of anything, and her friend told her she had to try it a few times to feel the effect. Fen, however, was not particularly curious, and did not try marijuana again until her first year in college. At the time, she was dating a student who smoked pot regularly, and she tried it again one night at a party with him. After inhaling deeply a few times and holding the smoke as she had seen him do, she began to feel cloudy, giggly, and quite hungry. Time seemed to move very slowly as well. She didn't feel particularly high, nor enthralled with what she did feel.

A year passed and Fen came upon the occasion of smoking pot for the third time in her life, amid a small gathering of friends, shortly before winter break. It was just a way of being sociable and joining the others. She smoked about one joint over the course of the evening and felt "very stoned," oddly detached from her body and from everything happening around her. "It wasn't a pleasant sensation," she recalls. "My head felt too present, and hollow somehow. I felt like my mind had somehow disconnected from my body. I didn't panic because I knew it was temporary. At least I thought it was." Fen remembers going to bed much later that evening thankful that she still had Saturday and Sunday ahead of her to get straight and study some for her midterms coming up the following week.

However, when she woke up the next morning she was feeling as strange and detached as the night before. Familiar objects around the room seemed somehow different in the morning light. Books, the alarm clock, a small trophy, a plant on the windowsill—they had all been there each day, but now they looked less familiar, as if she were seeing them for the first time. She told her boyfriend that she was still stoned, by now feeling frightened. The pot must have been stronger than usual, he said, assuring her not to worry because it would gradually dissipate over the course of the day. He was back to his normal self, however, which did not reassure Fen at all. She tried to relax her mind by having breakfast, listening to some music, and studying for her first exam. She found this terribly difficult to do, as it was very hard to focus on anything, and absorbed very little of what she was reading.

As the day unfolded, she felt she was in a dream, navigating through fog in slow motion, dazed and semi-aware of what was going on around her, time seeming eternal. She decided to go for a long walk, something that she often liked to do to relax whenever she felt stressed. She thought that the cold, fresh air might clear her head and help her feel more normal again—but it didn't. By bedtime that evening, Fen was starting to panic about her condition. She called several friends and her sister and asked them whether they had ever felt stoned and hung over from pot for so long. Although no one wanted to give her too straight an answer, she sensed that no one had.

By the next morning, Fen woke up to find that nothing had changed, and began to despair. In what turned out to be the most stressful few days of her life, she somehow managed to stick out her finals week, and returned home for the holidays. She then sobbingly confided to her parents what had happened to her. She now feared that she had somehow caused herself irreparable brain damage, and hated herself for having smoked. Although her family tried to comfort her by reminding her that she had done nothing different from many other good kids her age, she could not stop worrying that she had permanently damaged her brain and had only herself to blame.

After a couple weeks of no change, the family arranged for their doctor to see Fen. She tried to describe to him in detail exactly what she was feeling. He suggested that she was probably still stressed by the high demands of the semester that had just ended. She did not say anything, but Fen somehow knew this was not it. Although it had been a hard semester, she had been coping well with it, and she was not aware of feeling particularly stressed. She knew that this "physical" sensation had to be something different. She told the doctor that she was convinced the drug had somehow damaged her brain. To reassure her, he referred her to a neurologist.

Fen saw the new doctor, who ordered a few tests to make sure she was undamaged by her brief experiences with drugs. Both the magnetic resonance imaging (MRI) scan of her brain and the EEG test of her brain waves were normal. The neurologist then also told her that she appeared particularly stressed and anxious, and referred her to a psychiatrist. Meanwhile, there had been no change in the severity of Fen's symptoms for over a month now, and soon she had to return to school. She could not fathom going back and working hard with her head in a fog, a constant feeling that she was tripping or going insane. A few days later, she saw a psychiatrist, who told her that her experiences had a name, *depersonalization*. She had never heard of it and felt vastly relieved to find out that there was a name for what she was experiencing. The psychiatrist told her that the syndrome might have been triggered by her drug use and referred her to the psychiatry department of her school's university hospital.

Fen suffers from DDD; she has been experiencing unremitting dpdr for about five weeks without other psychological complaints, except for the secondary intense worrying about her condition. She is not clinically depressed, having panic attacks, or worrying extensively about anything other than her unusual and distressing experiences. She has developed, as often happens, intense obsessional ruminations surrounding her dpdr, but she does not have other obsessive-compulsive symptoms.

Does depersonalization triggered by marijuana always manifest itself as it did with Fen? Not always. While some people become "stoned" and then find that they can never seem to "sober up," others encounter an initial intense panic attack after smoking marijuana or hashish. This can be terrifying to a person who has never heard of such attacks or experienced any higher-than-normal degree of anxiety. This may happen after smoking just once, or after several times. Sometimes these panic attacks recur for several days, or even weeks, and then subside as the person settles into a classic state of chronic depersonalization. Does this mean that marijuana somehow caused irreversible brain damage to Fen's brain? No, there is no evidence for anything of this sort. Like any psychiatric condition, whether substance-induced or not, biological vulnerabilities are likely to play a role. That does not mean that the brain is permanently damaged, in the way that it may be in a neurological illness like stroke, for example. Rather it suggests that Fen's brain, and those of others like her, might have had some underlying neurochemical vulnerability that had previously laid dormant and unexpressed, only to be triggered by a particular drug (we will be discussing more about substance-triggered dpdr and the neurobiology of DDD in Chapters 6 and 8).

Did Fen really need an elaborate neurological work-up? Probably not. The sudden onset of her dpdr and its clear association to marijuana ingestion are classic, and have never been found to be associated with neurological lesions. When tests like brain scans or EEGs are done, they are usually looking for things like tumors and seizures. Fen's history is not suggestive of these, but her treating doctors were not particularly familiar with her symptoms. Yet other doctors conservatively err on the side of safety with any new-onset unusual psychiatric condition, wishing to ensure that nothing "medical" is going on. If Fen's dpdr had started more gradually, steadily increased over several months, and was associated with new-onset worsening headaches for example, a doctor would be much more inclined to do a neurological workup..

6

Refining the Diagnosis

Everything should be made as simple as possible, but not simpler.
—Albert Einstein

The human brain, the only organ capable of studying itself, has in the last two centuries turned its attention toward the mysterious phenomena of depersonalization and derealization, examining them from many perspectives. Depersonalization/derealization disorder (DDD) remains one of the most frequently misdiagnosed or underdiagnosed conditions in modern psychiatry. Why? Likely for several reasons. DDD is often accompanied by anxiety, depression, and other disorders, and patients may have trouble or hesitation expressing its vagaries in words that anyone but fellow sufferers can understand. A patient often winds up being treated for depression or anxiety even though they have tried to make clear that they were depressed *or* anxious only initially in their depersonalization course, or only well after their depersonalization had set in. And they feel less troubled by anxiety or depression compared to the dissociation.

Patients are often clear that what they are struggling most with is a sense of "unreality," "deadness," or "no self," and that they know the difference from being solely depressed or anxious. Clinicians, however, do not always agree, possibly because they have solid training in, and are therefore more comfortable dealing with, the domains of anxiety and depression. One telling distinction lies in how depersonalization/derealization (dpdr) symptoms fare alongside depression or anxiety symptoms. Does the person still feel quite depersonalized, even during periods when not anxious or depressed? If depression and anxiety wax and wane, does depersonalization follow along in tandem, or does it have "a life of its own"? We elaborated on all these considerations when diagnosing DDD in the previous two chapters.

Feeling Unreal. Second Edition. Daphne Simeon and Jeffrey Abugel, Oxford University Press. © Oxford University Press 2023. DOI: 10.1093/oso/9780197622445.003.0006

Epidemiology: Is DDD Rare?

To determine the "true" prevalence of any psychiatric, or for that matter medical, condition in the general population, a large "epidemiological" study is needed. Such a study randomly samples the population in different parts of a country, with well-established instruments and well-trained interviewers, so that the presence of various conditions can be detected and measured with accuracy. Such epidemiological studies have been conducted for all the major psychiatric disorders (mood disorders, anxiety disorders, psychotic disorders, posttraumatic stress disorder [PTSD], substance use disorders, etc.), but not for the dissociative disorders. Therefore, our estimates of their prevalence in the United States or elsewhere are, of necessity, more approximate, but still reliable.

The few studies that have looked at pathological dissociation in the general population have generated estimates in the range of 3% to 10%. The most reliable national estimate in the United States comes from the National Comorbidity Survey Replication study (NCS-R), which sampled 6,644 participants across the country in both urban and rural areas, and carefully accounted for sampling biases having to do with sociodemographic factors.[1] Though the survey did not ask questions diagnostic of the dissociative disorders, it included seven questions from the Dissociative Experiences Scale (DES, see Chapter 3) that capture the three domains of pathological dissociation (dpdr, amnesia, identity alteration).

Using a conservative cutoff, the study found that pathological dissociation likely indicative of a dissociative disorder had one-month national prevalence of 4.1%. This prevalence is naturally lower than lifetime prevalence, highlighting with greater certainty than ever that these disorders are not rare in the real world, but rather often go undetected or misdiagnosed. Furthermore, an algorithm (based on scores on the seven DES questions) was used to estimate the prevalence of the different dissociative disorders in the NCS-R, and estimated a 1.3% prevalence for a likely diagnosis of DDD.

Studies have also examined the prevalence of dpdr symptoms in population samples, and have reported rates in the broad range of 20% to 70%. In 2001, Dr. Aderibigbe and colleagues conducted a telephone survey in rural eastern North Carolina, inquiring about dpdr over a one-year period.[2] In the random sampling of 1,008 adults, it was found that 19% of the interviewees acknowledged depersonalization, 14% said they had experienced derealization, and nearly one-fourth (23%) reported having experienced both. This is quite a high rate for experiencing a psychiatric symptom over the course of a single year.

But before we begin calling North Carolina the "depersonalized state," a look at how the answers were assessed will shed some light on the results. People were asked the following question: "Sometimes people feel as though they are outside themselves, watching themselves do something; feel as if their body doesn't quite belong to them, like a robot; or feel like they are in a daze or a dream. Have you had any of these feelings within the last year?" A simple "yes" put 19% of the respondents into the depersonalized category. Similarly, to assess derealization the interviewees were asked: "Sometimes people feel as though other people or objects around them appear strange or changed in some way: that their surroundings are not quite real. Have you had any of these feelings in the last year?" As stated earlier, about 14% of the people called said "yes."

On average, the survey participants had experienced dpdr about 26 times over the course of the surveyed year, ranging from just one time to once a day. About one-fifth (19%) of the total sample had dpdr experiences that were defined as more substantial, lasting at least one hour or occurring at least three times. But was this all DDD? The answer is definitely not. For one, the very minimum of three hours in one year is not persistent enough to "qualify" for a disorder. Furthermore, dpdr experiences must cause significant distress or impairment to diagnose DDD. Also, the survey did not assess psychiatric symptoms other than dpdr, so it is not possible to know who of these people might have suffered from disorders like depression, anxiety disorders, PTSD, other dissociative disorders, or even no disorder at all. There is also the possibility that some may have been chronic substance users who were experiencing dpdr "under the influence." Asked when dpdr tended to happen, answers were as follows in decreasing order:

- when under severe stress (78%)
- when nervous or depressed (66%)
- when having upsetting memories of past events (45%)
- for no particular reason (35%)
- when in danger (25%)

These associations are nothing new and confirm what we already know about the contexts in which dpdr is most likely to occur. From the study, one can definitely infer that the one-year prevalence of DDD is much lower than the 19% with "more substantial" dpdr—but it cannot really tell us how much less. For example, those who dissociated when having disturbing memories were likely to be suffering from PTSD, or dissociative disorders other than DDD. Similarly, those who dissociated with danger, or under severe stress, might have been having an acute stress reaction, or at its more extreme "acute stress disorder," or again been suffering from another dissociative disorder, or from PTSD. Those having dissociation when anxious or depressed might have been suffering not from DDD but from the former.

It is then safe to say that some portion of the 35% who had dpdr "for no particular reason" were the "top" candidates for having DDD, assuming the symptoms were persistent or recurrent enough to constitute a disorder. Ultimately, even if only a portion (for the sake of an estimate, let's say one in three) of the 35% of the 19% of the total surveyed sample really suffered from DDD, we derive a very rough estimate of 2.2% for the disorder in this rural North Carolina population. Arrived at in such a different fashion, this approximate one-year DDD prevalence of 2.2% is very compatible with the one-month 1.4% prevalence for DDD-like disorder in the NCS-R national survey, established two decades later.[1]

The above estimates also concur with two community surveys carried out in the United Kingdom in the 1980s and again in the 1990s, which reported a 1.5% to 2% one-year prevalence of clinically significant dpdr, briefly assessed among many other symptoms.[3] Similarly, a nationally representative survey (using the ultra-brief two-item version, one dp and one dr question, of the Cambridge Depersonalization Scale, see Chapter 3) reported a prevalence of 1.9% for "clinically significant" dpdr, assessed for a 2-week period.[4] This survey also demonstrated (with a type of statistical analysis known as factor analysis) that dpdr constituted a distinct factor, separate from both depression and anxiety.

Dr. Colin Ross, a well-known expert in dissociative disorders, conducted a community survey of about 1,000 randomly selected inhabitants of Winnipeg, Canada, in the late 1980s. A dissociative experiences questionnaire was used for initial screening, followed by interviewing all those with elevated scores on the questionnaire.[5] Here it is important to note that conducting actual psychiatric interviews substantially strengthens the validity of any epidemiological study. The Canadian study yielded a 2.4% one-year prevalence for DDD. A more recent U.S. community study, conducted in New York State with diagnostic interviews, reported a lower 0.8% one-year prevalence for DDD.[6] Finally, a representative community-based study of women living in a city in central Turkey reported a 1.4% lifetime prevalence for DDD, highlighting that the disorder is not a "Western" phenomenon.[7]

In summary, then, and though we do not yet have a conclusive national study that used diagnostic interviewing for DDD, several studies reliably and compellingly converge around a 1% to 2% population prevalence for the disorder. That may sound like a small number in the scheme of things. But if you consider that the U.S. population stood at 330 million people in 2020, roughly 3.3 to 6.6 million people suffer from full-blown DDD. A 2% prevalence is double that of schizophrenia, and similar to the figures for bipolar disorder as well as for obsessive-compulsive disorder (OCD). Yet these other conditions are certainly more widely known and are granted considerably more attention and research funding.

Clinical Characteristics

Starting in the early 1990s, research centers in the United States and in the United Kingdom began to systematically investigate the characteristics of DDD through volunteer participants in their programs. In 2003, both centers published articles in leading journals describing the first large series of patients suffering from the disorder. The New York group's report, published in the *Journal of Clinical Psychiatry*, was based on a sampling of 117 consecutive patients suffering from depersonalization disorder according to the fourth edition of the *Diagnostic and Statistical Manual of Mental Disorders (DSM-IV)*.[8] The notion of "consecutive" is important here: all DDD participants seen by the research group over that time period were included—there was no pick-and-choosing, which could create biases by who was included and who was not. Each participant received an extensive in-person psychiatric interview. The London Institute of Psychiatry's report, published in the *British Journal of Psychiatry*, reported on 204 patients with chronic depersonalization; 124 were interviewed in person while the rest were assessed by phone or internet by completing a set of questionnaires.[9] In other words, the British study included participants who had clinical dpdr *symptoms*, of whom 71% were diagnostically confirmed to suffer from the disorder, whereas the American study only included participants actually diagnosed with DDD. A third study was published over a decade later, in 2016, by a German research group based in Mainz. This study included 223 patients with diagnosed DDD.[10]

Despite the somewhat different approaches and assessment tools used in the three studies, they transnationally spanned three "Western" countries and yielded strikingly similar findings, in most respects. Below we summarize these seminal findings about the disorder. Together, they offer a reliable and comprehensive profile of people with DDD, based on almost 550 cases combined. This number might not appear large, but it is tremendously respectable in the field of psychiatry for examining in great depth the characteristics of a previously uninvestigated disorder, traditionally assumed to be "rare." All three research centers studied adults with DDD, and gender distribution was very similar across the three studies, about 55% male. The U.S. study reported on whether men and women with DDD were in any way different: they were not, be it age of onset, course, duration, severity of symptoms, or co-occurring psychiatric disorders.[8]

The average DDD age of onset was 16 in the U.S. sample and 23 in the U.K. and German samples. Onset ranged from very early childhood, as far back as some people could remember, to late onset in a few people in their 40s, 50s, or 60s. Though the U.K. group found that those with earlier onset had more severe dpdr, the U.S. group did not replicate this finding. In the U.S. series, 80% cited onset by age 20 and 95% by age 25. In other words, this is very much a disorder of adolescence and early adulthood; onset in middle or late age is unusual. In translation, when people in their 30s seek treatment for DDD they are likely to have suffered from dpdr episodes for half of their lifetimes. Thankfully, it is our experience that since the first edition of this book, the spike in DDD research over the past 30 years, and the advent of social media, people are much likelier to self-identify their condition and to seek help in their early 20s. The people who participated in the early research studies had experienced DDD from as little as three months to as long as six decades.

The way DDD begins is highly variable. In some people it happens very suddenly, and these individuals typically recall the exact date, setting, and circumstances of how it started. For example, Bob will never forget the moment his dpdr set in, at age 20. The year had been very stressful, on a number of counts. His girlfriend of two years had broken up with him one month earlier. His grades had taken a plunge after his recent decision to pursue medicine and to take pre-med requirements. And, his mother had just been diagnosed with metastatic cancer. On the fateful morning of March 10, Bob was sitting in the packed chemistry classroom taking notes when he suddenly felt as if he were floating upwards. Everything seemed intensely unreal—the teacher looked like a robot, and Bob's scribbling hand felt disturbingly disconnected. He experienced a strange stillness, as if his ears were plugged, and he started to feel awfully strange in his own skin. He attributed his weird sensations to stress and fatigue and reassured himself they would go away when he'd go home and rest. However, he later woke up from a nap feeling just the same. He googled "unreal and disconnected," and the terms *depersonalization* and *derealization*, which he had not heard of before, readily popped up in his search. The labels reassured him some; at least what he was experiencing was a known entity with a name. This gave him the impetus to seek out help.

For others, the onset of dpdr can be insidious, setting in over a period of weeks or months. Less often, it may have started so far back that they really cannot recall how or when it came about (research shows about a 50/50 ratio of insidious vs. acute onset). Miriam, an only child, had a very hazy memory of her disturbing childhood. She had suddenly lost her mother to a car accident when she was five. Her father subsequently pulled away, soon remarried, and had two more children. Miriam was an outcast in the new family, a lonely and emotionally deprived child deeply longing to be seen and known by others. Her dpdr dated as far back as she could remember, and she has no recollections of her mother. Yet she'd always known that something felt "off" and strange, though she could not say exactly what. How did she know, if she could not recall a time when she felt "real"? Presumably, we all somehow "know," even without conscious memory or comparison, that there are other ways of feeling and being that may no longer be accessible. Perhaps it is instinct, remote implicit memory, or glimpses into what "being" is like during rare, fleeting moments of wakefulness, or even in dreams. Almost invariably, lifelong sufferers do seem to know the difference.

James, on the other hand, had never experienced depersonalization before he was 12. On the day when his beloved father gathered his three kids and announced that he was leaving their mother, James felt unreal for a few hours and then recovered. He vividly recalls feeling at the time that this must be a dream; it could not really be happening. Three years later, when he fractured his arm in a scary skiing accident, he felt depersonalized for two days. By the end of high school and early college, he began to experience longer bouts of depersonalization, lasting days or weeks, whenever he felt very stressed. Gradually and insidiously, before he knew it, the depersonalization "set in" for good. Looking back he thinks that it was probably sometime in the midst of his junior year in college that he no longer ever felt real.

The course of the disorder in over half of those who have it is continuous. Shockingly, such individuals are in a chronic dissociative state without a break. They may barely remember what it felt like not to be depersonalized and may refer to themselves as the "old me" versus the "new me," or as a "zombie," a "no self." In about one-third of people, the course of the disorder is episodic. In this scenario, dpdr comes and goes in episodes, lasting from days, to weeks, to months at a time, then subsiding until the next round. Although episodes can differ a lot from person to person, it is common for an episode to start abruptly yet to fade gradually. In about 10% of those with DDD, like James, the condition starts out with discrete dpdr episodes and over time the dpdr becomes continuous.

People with DDD often describe marked impairment in their daily living. The U.S., British, and German study took a close look at the important dimension of overall wellbeing in the disorder. In the American sample, despite solid education 13% of participants were unemployed and 14% were part-time employed. Many of those who were full-time employed described that their dpdr prevented them from having jobs that matched their intellectual capacity and training. Cognitive factors were often cited, such as difficulties with focusing, remembering, or being overstimulated by information (more on cognition in the next chapter). Those in more demanding jobs often felt that they were barely holding on, between the cognitive cloud that enveloped them and the intense preoccupation with dpdr symptoms and their implications. Sometimes, a sense of being phony and unworthy, of faking it all, plagues those with DDD. The U.S. study also found that only a minority of participants were involved in committed long-term relationships. Sadly, they described that within close relationships they often felt like they were just "going through the motions." Feelings were not readily accessible to them, and they experienced a pervasive sense of detachment and distance from their loved ones. It was not unusual for people to function better at work than in relationships.

The German study quantified impairment using a "global assessment of functioning" (GAF) measure. Strikingly, both work and social life impairment were greater in the DDD group than in the comparison group with depression; home life impairment was comparable in the two groups. GAF over the past year was rated, on average, at a low 55 in DDD (the range being 0 [worst] to 100 [best]). A GAF score between 50 and 60 reflects moderate to serious impairment in psychological, social, and occupational functioning. Roughly a third of DDD participants had scores below 50, traditionally considered a threshold for inpatient treatment, and one-fourth of the latter had received inpatient treatment over the past year.

Associations with Anxiety and Depressive Disorders

A wide range of depressive and anxiety disorders frequently exist alongside DDD. On a lifetime basis, the following disorders were present in the U.S. sample of 117 (overlapping): two-thirds had suffered from clinical, so-called "major," depression; one-third from dysthymia (chronic low-grade depression); one-third from social anxiety disorder, one-third from panic disorder, one-fifth from generalized anxiety disorder; and one-eighth from OCD. The German study found similarly high co-occurring disorders in DDD: 85% for depressive disorders, 43% for anxiety disorders, and 3% for OCD.

As we've already discussed, for a long time mainstream psychiatry had dismissed dpdr as a mere manifestation of underlying depressive or anxious conditions. When the U.S. study of 117 compared the age of onset of DDD to that of other coexisting disorders, no mood or anxiety disorder was found to have a significantly *earlier* age of onset than DDD—in fact, panic and depression started, on average, significantly *later* than DDD. This finding supports the conceptualization of dpdr as a *primary* rather than a secondary phenomenon. While the U.K. study did not compare age of onset of comorbid disorders, it did report that people with more severe depressive or anxiety symptoms also had more severe dpdr symptoms. This finding reflects that both depression and anxiety, when present, do tend to exacerbate dpdr symptoms as patients commonly describe.

Take Emma, for example. She first experienced depersonalization when she was 14, after her best friend died of a terminal illness. At 18 she left for college and first got depressed during her freshman year. Now, at age 34, she has endured two more episodes of clinical depression, as well as periods of milder depression. The dpdr never remitted during the two decades since its onset. Emma, like many other patients, can clearly describe the relationship between her depersonalization and depression symptoms. She states that in the first few years of depersonalization she simply did not feel depressed, despite how distraught she was over her sense of detachment from life. Later, every time he suffered from an episode of depression her depersonalization got worse; eventually the depression would lift, while the depersonalization only returned to its usual baseline. She describes it in this way: "The depression makes it worse, but the depersonalization is always there: they don't just go hand in hand with each other."

Associations with PTSD

A diagnosis of PTSD requires the occurrence of a major traumatic event, an event that is threatening to a person's life or integrity and that a patient can describe as preceding and precipitating the onset of their symptoms. By most standards these are events that are horrific and overwhelming, such as combat, rape, assault, natural disasters, terrorist attacks, and severe childhood maltreatment. These kinds of incidents are known to cause PTSD in large numbers of previously unaffected people—at least 25% of those exposed to such traumas.

People with DDD show a low (5% or less) lifetime prevalence of PTSD. This appears to be a function of the different magnitude and quality of the traumas with which DDD tends to be associated, which are typically less extreme and life-threatening. This low rate of PTSD in those with DDD is in sharp contrast to the more "severe" dissociative disorders, such as dissociative identity disorder, which is associated with high rates of PTSD. In this sense, chronic depersonalization offers a unique research model for better understanding the different preexisting vulnerabilities, types of trauma, and pathogenetic pathways that lead to pathological dissociation versus posttraumatic stress presentations.

Importantly, with the advent of the *DSM-5* a new subtype of PTSD was introduced, based on extensive research and evidence[11]: the "dissociative subtype." The criteria for this subtype require clinically significant dpdr, just like in DDD. Of course, in this case the diagnosis made is one of dissociative PTSD, not DDD. Individuals with this subtype of PTSD tend to have childhood trauma histories, again highlighting the relationship between early adversity and later pathological dissociation. Though DDD and PTSD are readily distinct, the delineation of this new PTSD subtype has now brought dpdr more to the forefront of clinicians' awareness. This is a hopeful development, as clinicians who become increasingly familiar with assessing and treating dpdr in other contexts will also be more open to a DDD diagnosis, when it applies.

Associations with Personality Disorders

Regarding what psychiatry calls personality disorders (longstanding personality styles that are pervasive and dysfunctional), only the U.S. case series examined and diagnostically assessed their presence in DDD. No single personality disorder was uniquely or strongly associated with DDD; rather, the whole range of personality disorders was widely represented among the DDD participants. The three most common personality disorders were:

- *Avoidant* (23%): These are people who are overly self-conscious in social settings, are frightened to make overtures to others, and tend to be shy and reclusive.
- *Borderline* (21%): These are people who exhibit instability in their mood and behaviors, tend to be impulsive, are often angry, and lack a well-formed sense of identity.
- *Obsessive-compulsive* (21%): These are people who are overly perfectionistic, detail-oriented, rigid, and controlling.

All the other personality disorders were represented as well, such as paranoid, narcissistic, dependent, histrionic, schizotypal, and schizoid. About 40% of the patients did *not* have a diagnosable personality disorder. Not surprisingly, DDD patients who had a more severe personality disorder (e.g., borderline or narcissistic, associated with disturbances in self cohesion and identity consolidation) had more severe dissociative symptoms than the remaining sample.

What Precipitates Chronic Dpdr?

As with any psychiatric disorder, a foremost question can be: what brought it on? Why did it happen at all, and why did it happen when it did? DDD, like other mental illness, likely involves genetic predispositions, followed by early life events that enhance vulnerability, followed by later stressors, often traumatic ones, that eventually trigger the onset of chronic clinical symptoms. Unlike some of the better-studied mental disorders, less is known about these components when it comes to DDD, yet our knowledge continues to increase.

Heritability

When questioned informally, only a few people (5% in the U.S. series and 10% in the U.K. series) described some known family history of depersonalization, while the German study did not report on dpdr family history; relatives were not formally interviewed in any of the three studies. Does this mean that there is no heritable component to dpdr? Not necessarily. Firstly, it's quite likely that prior generations simply didn't know what to call their symptoms or were too ashamed to discuss them—even today we remain struck by the number of patients who have not shared their condition with those close to them. Perhaps more importantly, a familial heritable component for dpdr may rest not in dpdr experiences per se, but rather in a more general propensity for dissociating.

One of the ways to study "heritability" is to examine identical versus non-identical (fraternal) twins. In effect, the "difference" in how often a condition occurs in both members of identical versus non-identical twin pairs reflects the condition's "genetic" heritable component. Three studies, so far, have examined the heritability of dissociation, though not dpdr per se. Two of these behavioral genetic studies, as they are known, reported conflicting findings; they both measured dissociative symptoms in twins using the Dissociative Experiences Scale. While one study found no heritable component to pathological dissociation,[12] the other study reported an approximately 50% genetic component, 55% for normative dissociation and 48% for pathological dissociation[13] (see Chapter 3 for the distinction between the two). The genetic correlation between normative and pathological dissociation was strong, suggesting that common genetic factors underlie the capacity for both types of dissociation, and that the pathological (nurture) builds on the normative (nature) when life circumstances occur that promote pathology. The non-genetic heritability component was attributable to nonshared environmental influences, meaning life experiences unique to each twin within a pair.

A third genetic study examined dissociation in middle childhood and adolescent children who were either fraternal twins or full versus adoptive siblings.[14] Children were rated by both parents and teachers for dissociative-like behaviors using a well-established measure. The study found that individual differences in dissociation were quite stable over time, supporting the scientific belief that dissociation is not just a temporary state of mind, but also a trait that variably and stably characterizes different individuals. The study reported substantial amounts of both genetic and nonshared environmental contributions (like the above-mentioned study of adult twins[13]) but negligible shared environmental contributions.

Taken together, studies suggest that dissociation is a "trait diathesis:" an inherent predisposition, be it strength or vulnerability, that some individuals possess more than others. When adversity hits, be it from the very early years to much later, pathology builds on normality and strikes. Frank Putnam,[15] a leading authority on dissociation, has proposed that the very discrete behavioral states of newborns become gradually integrated over time with smooth and seamless transitions between states, as a young child learns to self-regulate and forms an increasingly cohesive sense of self, in the presence and with the help of a good-enough caregiver. When this normative developmental process is hampered, a child may remain inordinately compartmentalized or detached surrounding painful experiences, in effect dissociative, and the foundations are laid for pathological dissociation and its related disorders.

The idea that people with DDD possess an in-place predisposition toward dissociation is perhaps supported by the personal stories that they sometimes relay. Some remember fleeting moments of depersonalization from a very early age, way before the disorder set in with any severity or permanence. Some may not even recall passing instances of dpdr symptoms per se, but rather a willingness, ease, or readiness, a propensity to detach themselves from disturbing happenings around them. With the preexisting diathesis in place, something may eventually happen to trigger the actual onset of a clinical condition. These triggers vary in different people with DDD and are discussed later on in this chapter.

Psychological Precipitants

In the U.S. sample, 25% of all people reported onset during a period of severe stress, 12% with panic attacks, and 9% with depression. Similarly, in the British sample 15% reported onset with a "psychological" trigger while 14% reported onset with a "traumatic event." Any overwhelming and disturbing mental state can trigger dpdr in an individual with a dissociative diathesis and other preexisting vulnerabilities (see next chapter), and the dpdr may then become persistent and take on "a life of its own." A precipitating event can threaten the very integrity of the sense of self and induce a profound, anguished state of "who am I?" This shift sets off depersonalization that over time may become autonomous from the precipitating state.

When dpdr is initially triggered by an episode of another psychiatric disorder, like depression or panic, sufferers are particularly likely to be misdiagnosed and have their symptoms "dismissed" as part-and-parcel of the other condition. Surprisingly, this often happens even when patients clearly describe that the symptoms of depression or panic (the two most common culprits) are long gone, and that they are distinctly aware of now suffering from something very different. DDD patients often become demoralized and hopeless about their condition when one practitioner after the other tells them that the dpdr is just another symptom of their depression or anxiety and should be treated (typically unsuccessfully) as such. In this sense, the onset of chronic dpdr in the context of another more common and better-known psychiatric condition presents a tricky challenge for accurate diagnostic dissection.

Severe stress was another commonly reported precipitant for chronic dpdr—one-fourth of DDD participants, as previously mentioned, in the U.S. sample. Although these stressors may or may not be of a magnitude meriting the characterization "traumatic" in the minds of some, they may well be traumatic for the individuals undergoing them. Traumatic stress of all sorts can trigger DDD. Some people describe prolonged struggles with troubled marriages and difficult divorces, major life transitions such as leaving home for college or finishing college and entering the workforce, pregnancy and the early postpartum period of being with a newborn. Even extremely demanding work conditions that lead to "burnout" can be a trigger.

Why a stressful life event may prove particularly overwhelming for certain people can be quite mysterious and not apparent to the untrained observer. For example, Lisa entered chronic depersonalization when she found out that Debbie, the sister of her best friend, had committed suicide. This was, of course, tragic, but most people would not become chronically depersonalized like Lisa. It is always necessary to look closely at the personal event and the very specific symbolic meanings that it may have had for a particular individual, to truly appreciate the severity of symptoms to which it led. For Lisa, further exploration revealed that she had experienced intense and prolonged guilt over Debbie's suicide. Debbie had been very fond of Lisa and had repeatedly tried to befriend and confide in her. Lisa had consistently rebuffed Debbie, not only out of a sense of loyalty to her best friend but because Debbie was younger, less cool, and outright unpopular. After the suicide, Lisa was left feeling somehow responsible, doubting her prior stance toward Debbie and regretting that she never really got to know her, or try to help her.

Early childhood adversity (which we discuss in the next chapter) and later stressful events have powerful and complex interactions in precipitating all kinds of psychiatric pathology. Extensive research has shown how potent this interaction can be across a variety of disorders. Compared to a person who did not experience childhood adversity, a person who had a traumatic childhood is "set up" to be more vulnerable to challenges and stressors that happen later on, and is more likely to develop symptoms of any sort, be it anxiety, depression, posttraumatic stress, dpdr, psychosis, addiction, or whatever else they may be biologically vulnerable to. Then again, it is also important to remember that childhood adversity does not always lead to later pathology. Some people are unusually resilient to the impacts of trauma, and the factors, whether biological or psychosocial, that contribute to such resilience are as important to understand as the factors associated with pathology.

The German study took a close look at psychosocial stressors and quantified them in the DDD sample. The study assessed 20 common stressors over the past month, and a stressor was rated as positive if an individual said that they were bothered "a lot" by it. Endorsement by the DDD group, from highest to lowest (overlapping), was as follows:

- worrying about health (62%)
- having no one to turn to when having a problem (29%)
- stress at work or at school (28%)
- weight or appearance (27%)
- financial problems or worries (25%)
- little or no desire or pleasure in sex (24%)
- caretaker stress—children, parents, or other family (22%)
- thinking/dreaming about a terrible happening (19%)
- difficulties with romantic partner (19%)
- something bad happened recently (13%)

The cumulative stressor burden over the past month was 7.7 out of 20 stressors in the DDD group, undeniably notable. Endorsing that, on average, nearly eight recent life situations were very bothersome is no small matter, and of course in a clinical setting would merit thorough exploration. Yet, interestingly so, the DDD patients as a group were less bothered by these stressors than the comparison group with depression (this group's cumulative score was 9.7). The researchers were intrigued by this finding and wondered whether DDD patients are "often unable to consider psychological problems and interpersonal conflicts as relevant causes," especially as they tend to be highly preoccupied by the seeming physicality of their symptoms and on a quest for physical explanations and causes. Indeed, the very high endorsement of "worrying about health" (see above) likely reflects this pre-occupation. The difficulty that DDD patients often have with making mean-ingful psychological connections between their state of mind and important life experiences is a hallmark of the condition, and one that clinicians are very familiar with—we will be discussing this more in later chapters.

Paradoxically there are occasions when dpdr is precipitated by posi-tive experiences. A classic example from the annals of psychoanalysis is Freud's visit to the Acropolis, which we talked about in Chapter 2. One DDD patient's history involved a highly disturbing home life when he was a child. Deshawn's father had a severe personality disorder and was a very troubled and preoccupied man, a drinker as well, who made life miserable for those around him. Deshawn grew up feeling "unseen" by his father; they never spent time together or did any of the fun guy stuff that his friends did with their dads. In addition, Deshawn was often walking on eggshells at home, un-sure of when his father would explode and start ranting in the long evenings after dinner. Robert's mom was kind but passive, and much closer to her older child, Deshawn's sister. Deshawn was finally accepted to the prestigious college at the top of his list, where he made many new friends, met a young woman, and enjoyed learning. Yet, when at long last he was able to leave be-hind him the miseries of his home, he was thrust into a state of chronic dpdr. Perhaps he was so deprived that he couldn't tolerate such intense positive feelings and experiences—they were new to him, and unsafe. Or maybe he felt disbelief that his new life was "for real" and feared he would lose it all. Or maybe he felt ashamed for hardly caring about how his parents were doing back home. Or maybe he simply didn't know how to contain the previously unknown sense of excitement and hope, regulate it, and integrate it with his usual perceptions of who he was.

Deshawn's case makes the point that what is overwhelming for one person may not be overwhelming for the next, because all that we experience in the world is processed internally and is heavily laden with unique personal meanings. The bottom line is that overwhelming experience of any sort can trigger persistent dpdr in those who have an underlying propensity to dissociate, often coupled with vulnerabilities related to earlier adversity—whether the bearer of the experience knows it or not.

DDD Precipitated by Drugs

One well-known DDD precipitant is drug ingestion, even when drug use has not been habitual. At times, even one-time use can throw an individual into a chronic depersonalized state. Nowadays, this is frequently described by people who post their personal stories on internet websites or participate in some of the discussion forums found within these sites. These are not cases of a straightforward, short-lived reaction or "high" from the drug—the dpdr persists long after the drug's direct influence is gone.

The first reports of isolated cases of chronic depersonalization induced by cannabis came out back in the 1980s.[16,17] Nearly two decades later, the U.S. and the U.K. studies addressed this issue methodically and provided detailed figures. In both cohorts, a substantial minority of DDD cases were drug-triggered in onset. In the U.S. cohort of 117 DDD patients, 22% of all participants reported that drugs precipitated the disorder, about 13% (of the total group) for cannabis, 6% for hallucinogens, 2% for Ecstasy, and 1% for ketamine.[8] The U.K. cohort yielded a strikingly close figure: 24% of participants identified drugs as precipitating the disorder, about 12% (of the total group) for cannabis, 2% for Ecstasy, 1% for LSD, 1% for ketamine, and 8% for combinations involving at least one of the aforementioned drugs.[18] Though the drug-induced DDD group was younger and had a male preponderance, the drug-induced and non–drug-induced DDD groups were otherwise strikingly similar. In other words, it is important to realize that regardless of precipitant, the condition is the same and unfolds in the same ways. Of note, the German study did not report on the matter of drug use as a precipitant of DDD.[10]

The largest study to date comparing drug-induced versus non–drug-induced chronic dpdr was published in 2009 and consisted of an anonymous internet survey of 394 individuals.[19] The two groups were just about equal in number of participants and had similar scores on the Cambridge Depersonalization Scale. And the two groups were clinically very similar in all regards, though the drug-induced group reported greater (though not major) spontaneous improvement in dpdr with time. Quite a bit was uncovered about the drug-related history of the 196 participants in the drug-induced group. Importantly, during the ingestion that induced chronic symptoms, a very large majority of participants, 87%, endorsed having had a "bad trip."

By far the two most common single-drug ingestions in the drug-induced group were cannabinoids (45%) and hallucinogens (13%), followed by Ecstasy (4%), and single cases of ketamine, salvia, and a general anesthetic. In the one-third of the drug-induced group that had taken more than one drug, the drugs typically involved in single-drug ingestions figured in a similar way. The lifetime drug history of participants in the drug-induced group, prior to dpdr onset, was quite telling. Regarding marijuana, roughly one-third had taken it very sporadically, 10 or fewer times; one-third had taken it more frequently (11 to 100 times); another third were more habitual users (100 to 500 times). About two-thirds became depersonalized immediately, during the high, and a large majority (70%) never used marijuana again subsequent to dpdr onset. Regarding hallucinogens, a two-thirds majority had done them 10 or fewer times, and the onset of dpdr was reported as somewhat more protracted after the ingestion, within one week for most participants. As with cannabinoids, about 70% never took a hallucinogen again after dpdr set in. Of the eight participants with Ecstasy-induced dpdr, six of the eight had never tried it before, and half never used it again. In brief, then, drug-induced DDD need not involve, and often does not involve, habitual or problematic drug use, and the resulting dissociation is disturbing and aversive enough that most will not use the culprit drug again.

Some major drug groups, illicit or prescribed, that have *not* been implicated in inducing chronic dpdr are opiates, like heroin and painkillers; stimulants, like the amphetamines and cocaine; and benzodiazepines. Alcohol also does not appear to trigger dpdr, nor to typically exacerbate it, except with chronic and heavy use that is associated with a feeling of detachment and fogginess akin to a hangover. Alcohol is, however, known to potentially exacerbate both depression or anxiety, and in this way may more indirectly fuel dpdr. In other words, the types of drugs implicated in inducing DDD are specific and consistent, and this fact may have neurobiological implications (more on this follows in Chapter 8).

How do people go into this high and never come out of it? They wake up the next morning and find themselves in a different state of mind that doesn't ease up and in which they may remain stuck for months or years. One possible answer, just mentioned, is that a very specific chemical trigger has tipped something off balance in the brain of a person who is already biologically vulnerable, and that this neurochemical change manifests itself in the form of depersonalization. Other explanations for drug-triggered onsets are also plausible. The actual experience of the "high," especially after the "bad trip" that is typical in these scenarios, could be so terrifying and overwhelming to the self's usual sense of constancy and cohesion that it throws some people into a protracted altered state.

One clinical example of this involved a patient, Mary, who had an intense phobia of death. There were many instances in her life in which she behaved "counterphobically"—that is, she deliberately approached this fear by taking risks, attempting to master and overcome it. Her fear was likely related to a near-drowning experience that occurred when she was five, as vivid in her memory now as it had been many years ago. When she used Ecstasy, she encountered the idea of death in vivid hallucinations and was terrified. She depersonalized and then did not come out of this altered state. So, it can be hard to know whether the triggering event was chemical, psychological, or both.

More about Marijuana

The active ingredient in marijuana is known as tetrahydrocannabinol (THC), a psychoactive substance that produces the "high" associated with smoking marijuana or hashish. The chemical structure of THC is similar to the brain's own ("endogenous") cannabinoid, anandamide. Endogenous cannabinoids such as anandamide are neurotransmitters, sending chemical messages between neurons (brain nerve cells) and thus impacting brain areas involved in pleasure, memory, thinking, concentration, movement, coordination, sensations, and time perception. Because of its similarity to anandamide, THC can attach to the brain's endogenous cannabinoid receptors and activate them, disrupting a wide range of mental and physical functions. This neural communication network, known as the endocannabinoid system, plays a critical role in various aspects of normal functioning, so interfering with it can have profound effects.[20]

Cannabinoid receptors are abundant throughout the brain, especially in the hypothalamus, the hippocampus, and the amygdala, the ancient part of the brain responsible for primal emotions, including fear. With cannabis rich in THC, the brain suddenly receives more cannabinoids than usual. This cannabinoid excess can overstimulate the amygdala, resulting a fear reaction of heightened anxiety or panic that, in turn, may trigger depersonalization in susceptible individuals.[21]

So many people casually smoke marijuana—how common is it for it to trigger chronic depersonalization? It is not common, but it is well-established to occur. Given the very high prevalence of marijuana use in the general population, an outcome of chronic depersonalization is infrequent. Still, it happens often enough for specialist clinicians to be quite familiar with this presentation and history. Online forums and websites paint the picture of drug-induced chronic dpdr with raw immediacy. Of 200 personal stories compiled by www.depersonalization.info between 2000 and 2010, 30% implicated pot or hash as the identifiable source of onset, pretty close to the 23% cited by the two DDD cohorts reported in 2003.[8,18] Ages ranged from the teens to the 50s. Many accounts described acute panic attacks that were then followed by lasting dpdr. The postings described consistently similar dpdr symptoms, and about 10% of stories attested to periodic feelings of depersonalization prior to smoking pot, usually in early childhood.

With marijuana now legal in many states in the United States, more potent that it was decades ago and available to ingest in various forms and strengths, it would not be surprising if future research reveals an increase in the prevalence of drug-induced DDD. We are already seeing in clinical practice patients with chronic dpdr triggered by legally purchased marijuana, especially with high-potency edibles, so this is an unfolding story early in its making.

Preliminary studies examining the impact of legalization have already documented wider (and often perceived as safer) marijuana use, increasing emergency room visits related to cannabis, an increase in cannabis use disorder, though not in psychotic disorders so far, and a greater proportion of users with personality disorders in the post-legalization period.[22,23] Many more studies will undoubtedly be coming our way in the 2020s. The matter of legalization and its impact on mental illness extends well beyond DDD and poses the larger question of which psychiatric disorders unrestricted cannabis has the potential to precipitate or exacerbate and, conversely, whether unrestricted use might prove helpful in other psychiatric disorders. In the nascent field of the impact of legalized marijuana on mental illness, for now there is limited preliminary evidence for a positive impact on social anxiety, sleep disorders, PTSD, and attention-deficit/hyperactivity disorder (ADHD), though much more research is needed.[24] How will our societies strike an optimal balance, unbiased by financial profit and other incentives?

Marijuana's therapeutic usefulness in some medical conditions like intractable chronic pain, epilepsy, and cancer is already indisputable; psychiatry is more complicated, and the bigger story of marijuana and medicine is just beginning to unfold.

DDD Clinical Profile, Part I

- Average age of onset is in adolescence or late adolescence/young adulthood.
- Men and women are about equally affected.
- The disorder causes great distress and dysfunction.
- Onset can be acute or insidious.
- Dpdr symptoms more often become continuous over time but may remain episodic.
- Normative dissociation, and by extension a vulnerability to pathological dissociation, carries a heritable component.
- There is substantial comorbidity with mood or anxiety disorders, but none of these disorders has a unique relationship to DDD.
- Personality disorders are common, but no personality disorder is uniquely associated with DDD.
- The most common precipitants of DDD are severe stressors, episodes of other mental illness, and drug ingestions. In a sizable portion of cases there is no readily identifiable precipitant.
- The two most common drugs that induce DDD are cannabis and hallucinogens. Most users are casual rather than habitual and avoid the culprit drug after the onset of lasting dpdr.

Part II of this DDD Clinical Profile is in the next chapter.

7

Trauma, Attachment, Emotion, and Cognition

[since feeling is first]

—E. E. Cummings

In the previous chapter we examined more proximal events that commonly precipitate the onset of depersonalization/derealization disorder (DDD), whether it be the first clinical depersonalization/derealization (dpdr) episode or any subsequent one. Here we shift our focus to the broader lifetime vulnerabilities that render an individual more likely to manifest DDD. These essentially have to do with the "make-up" of a person—their history of adversity from early on in life, as well as the ways in which they process experience, emotionally and cognitively.

Childhood Trauma

A history of childhood maltreatment is quite common in those with mental illnesses of all sorts, markedly more so than in those without. This basic fact has been indisputably established and replicated over and over in psychiatry, through large-scale epidemiological studies of the past quarter-century that leave no room for doubt. In fact, it has been shown that the impact of adverse childhood experiences (ACEs) on adult mental health is *dosed* and *cumulative*. ACE studies use a comprehensive index of childhood maltreatment that combines abuse and neglect (i.e., physical abuse, emotional abuse, sexual abuse, physical neglect, emotional neglect, witnessing domestic violence) and is supplemented by adverse experiences related to "household

Feeling Unreal. Second Edition. Daphne Simeon and Jeffrey Abugel, Oxford University Press. © Oxford University Press 2023. DOI: 10.1093/oso/9780197622445.003.0007

dysfunction" and not directly "targeting" the child (e.g., parental loss, discord, substance abuse, mental illness, incarceration).

Starting with the landmark Centers for Disease Control–Kaiser Permanente ACE study of 1998,[1] ACEs have been found to be *common* in the general population, with about two-thirds of all adults having experienced at least one. As the number of ACE events climbs, the association with adverse outcomes in adulthood becomes quite striking and follows a *dose-response* pattern—mental illnesses, chronic physical ailments, high morbidity (decreased life potential), and even mortality (premature death). In fact, childhood maltreatment has been associated, in this dose-response fashion, with many psychiatric disorders: schizophrenia, bipolar disorder, depressive and anxiety disorders, posttraumatic stress disorder (PTSD), and, of course, dissociative disorders.

The most recent edition of the *Diagnostic and Statistical Manual of Mental Disorders* (*DSM-5-TR*) summarizes the relationship between dissociative disorders and trauma as follows:[2]

> "Dissociative disorders are frequently found in the aftermath of a wide variety of psychologically traumatic experiences in children, adolescents, and adults."
> "'[T]raumatic experiences' refers to experiences that result in psychological sequelae."
> "Therefore, in *DSM-5*, the dissociative disorders are placed next to, but are not part of, the trauma- and stressor-related disorders, reflecting the close relationship between these diagnostic classes."

It further states: "Across cultural contexts, risk factors for dissociative pathology include earlier onset of trauma; neglect and sexual, physical, and emotional abuse by parents; cumulative early life trauma and adversities; and repeated sustained trauma or torture associated with captivity."

The above was compellingly demonstrated through an analysis of the National Comorbidity Survey–Replication (NCS-R) database, which gathered mental illness statistics across the entire U.S. population (see epidemiology section of the previous chapter). The article, published in 2022 in the *Journal of Trauma and Dissociation*, examined the relationships between adulthood pathological dissociation and history of childhood maltreatment.[3] It was found that "total" childhood maltreatment powerfully predicted the current severity of pathological dissociative symptoms in the adults who partook in the national survey. Total childhood trauma also *specifically* predicted the severity of *each* of the three major types of pathological dissociative experiences (dpdr, amnesia, and identity alteration). Furthermore, *each* of the childhood maltreatment categories predicted pathological dissociation severity *uniquely and additively*, in the fashion just described for cumulative ACE events.

In the NCS-R survey, childhood maltreatment in the group with pathological dissociation was, in fact, significantly greater than in those with lifetime histories of major depression (except for emotional neglect, which was comparable) and similar to those with lifetime histories of PTSD. The categories of childhood maltreatment that were examined by this study included physical abuse, witnessing domestic violence, physical neglect, emotional abuse, and emotional neglect. Sexual abuse data were not available to the authors, rendering the findings even more remarkable, as this type of maltreatment comprises a sine qua non of DID.

Childhood maltreatment has been investigated in DDD, and studies have now consistently documented that emotional maltreatment (abuse and/or neglect) is the predominant type of childhood trauma. Other types of childhood maltreatment do occur but are, on the whole, less typical and distinguishing. The first study examining childhood interpersonal trauma in DDD was published about two decades ago by the U.S. group, in the prestigious *American Journal of Psychiatry*.[4] A group of 49 adults with DDD was compared to a healthy control group without lifetime psychiatric diagnoses (but not prescreened with regard to trauma). A detailed childhood trauma interview was used that takes about an hour to administer and measures six categories of childhood trauma:

- Separations and losses
- Physical neglect
- Emotional abuse
- Physical abuse
- Sexual abuse
- Witnessing domestic violence

Of the six categories, three—emotional abuse, physical abuse, and sexual abuse—were scored significantly higher in DDD. Of these three, further extensive analyses revealed that *emotional abuse* alone stood out as the one more specific type of maltreatment intimately related to DDD. The *average* emotional abuse scores in the DDD group reflected frightening experiences—yelling and screaming by caretakers, threats like "I'll kill you," or statements like "I wish I'd never had you." The emotional abuse occurred frequently, setting the emotional tone while growing up for years on end. It involved both parents in about half of DDD cases, the mother only in 12, and the father only in nine.

Emotional abuse started earlier in life in the DDD group, on average at the young age of five. The "total" emotional abuse score predicted the severity of current dpdr—simply put, the earlier, more frequent, and more severe the emotional abuse, the stronger the association with the disorder. This hallmark study demonstrated that pervasive emotional maltreatment, without respite or shelter from either parent, creates a damaging and dangerous emotional environment wherein a child prone to dissociation may start to emotionally detach out of fright long before clinical dpdr sets in. It is as if "nothing terrible is really happening." This is often reflected in the initial history-taking with DDD patients, who tend to minimize and de-affectualize their past experiences.

The second component of childhood emotional maltreatment is *emotional neglect*. Emotional neglect consists of experiences leading a child to feel unloved, unsupported, and ignored in their emotional needs and wants. The caretaker may not care to know, or have the capacity to know, how the child feels. In more recent years, the pervasive and damaging role of neglect has received increasing attention across psychiatric disorders. It is rather common for DDD patients to recall that, as children, they received little positive parenting: caring, involvement, physical warmth and affection, nurturance, support, guidance, and appropriate socialization. When a parent is not emotionally available, other negative experiences of the child are more likely to remain unprocessed, to build and fester. Emotional deprivation can have profound lifelong consequences, as it inhibits the development of a genuine, positive sense of self—there is an intimate relationship between emotion, experiencing, and identity formation.

The childhood trauma interview reported on in the original study importantly did *not* include an assessment of *neglect*, either emotional or physical. Later studies used an easier-to-administer measure of childhood trauma, the 25-item self-report Childhood Trauma Questionnaire (CTQ).[5] The CTQ covers five maltreatment categories: emotional abuse, physical abuse, sexual abuse, physical neglect, and emotional neglect. Each category contains five questions, scored from 1 to 5. Not surprisingly, but nonetheless reassuringly, this short questionnaire and the earlier lengthy interview were in very strong agreement in one DDD study that used both.[6]

Over the past two decades, the CTQ has become established as the most widely used measure of childhood maltreatment. Researchers have examined it on a larger scale and have developed a "clinically recommended" cutoff score for each of its five maltreatment categories, reliably associated with psychiatric and medical sequelae and translating into higher healthcare costs.[7] Childhood maltreatment costs not only the child, but the society as well. The U.S. group went back to their original data sets and re-examined CTQ findings across several studies, while applying these recommended cutoffs. In this way, it was possible to calculate the prevalence of "clinically significant" childhood trauma in a larger sample of 93 patients with DDD, 48 women and 45 men, with an average age of 31.[8] The results put concrete numbers on the problem of maltreatment in the disorder, which did *not* differ by gender. In decreasing order, the prevalence of clinically meaningful childhood trauma was as follows:

- **Emotional abuse:** 49% (called names by family; parents wished was never born; felt hated by family; family said hurtful things; was emotionally abused)
- **Physical neglect:** 40% (not enough to eat; not taken care of; parents drunk or high; wore dirty clothes; not taken to the doctor)
- **Emotional neglect:** 36% (didn't feel loved; wasn't made to feel important; wasn't looked out for; family didn't feel close; family wasn't a source of strength)
- **Physical abuse:** 27% (hit hard enough to see doctor; hit hard enough to leave bruises; punished with hard objects; was physically abused; hit badly enough to be noticed)
- **Sexual abuse:** 20% (was touched sexually; hurt if didn't do something sexual; made to do sexual things; was molested; was sexually abused)

At least one clinically significant type of trauma occurred in nearly two-thirds (63%)—put conversely, only a *minority* of DDD patients had *no* notable history of maltreatment. A history of *emotional maltreatment* in the form of either abuse or neglect was present in 55% of patients, the majority. A history of *pervasive emotional maltreatment*, meeting cutoffs for both abuse and neglect, was present in nearly one-third of the DDD group (30%). *Pervasive neglect*, physical and emotional, was present in about one-fourth of patients (26%). Lastly, patients meeting clinical significance for *all five* traumas approached one in 10 (9%). It is readily evident that, taken together, these numbers are quite striking, and settle any lingering questions or doubts regarding the common and important contribution of maltreatment to the genesis of DDD.

The British research group has not systematically pursued the investigation and implications of childhood maltreatment in DDD over the years, compelled by a more cognitive and anxiety-centered perspective. However, one of the group's key investigators has made note of the potential significance of childhood trauma, in relation to emotional processing difficulties and neurobiological underpinnings (see later in this chapter and next chapter).[9]

On the other hand, the German research group has taken interest in depersonalization and childhood trauma and reported relevant findings in two separate studies—a DDD clinical study as well as a larger epidemiological study. The CTQ was used in a series of 223 patients with diagnosed DDD,[10] and the study reported the average scores for each of the five trauma categories, which turned out to be very similar to those found across the ocean in New York in the DDD sample just described—arguably, we can have confidence in the confluence of numbers. The German investigators appeared to underplay the significance of their findings, emphasizing that childhood trauma in DDD was no greater than in the study's comparison group of people with depression. However, there is another way of thinking about this similarity to depression. Not only is depression known to be powerfully associated with childhood trauma in a sizable portion of sufferers, but there also is an extensive literature demonstrating that, in the presence of childhood trauma, the treatment of depression with medication alone and *without psychotherapy* is not effective enough. In 2020, renowned depression researchers Drs. Elizabeth Lippard and Charles Nemeroff titled a telling and important paper on this matter "The Devastating Clinical Consequences of Child Abuse and Neglect: Increased Disease Vulnerability and Poor Treatment Response in Mood Disorders," emphasizing the lasting psychological and biological impacts of childhood maltreatment.[11]

The second German study was a nationwide survey of about 1,300 adults, in which dpdr was quantified via nine questions from the Cambridge Depersonalization Scale and, when present, was rated as "clinically significant" or "some impairment."[12] A brief parental rearing questionnaire was also given, asking about three dimensions of a child's emotional experience when growing up (rejection and punishment; emotional warmth; and con-trol and overprotection), separately assessed for each of the two parents. It turned out that both "clinically significant" and "some impairment" dpdr were associated with increased *rejection and punishment* from *both* parents while growing up. Participants with "some impairment" additionally re-ported experiencing greater *control* and *overprotection*, by *both* parents. This survey provided further compelling support for the link between emotional maltreatment and dpdr on a community-based scale, again highlighting the frequent involvement of both parents,[4] and neatly converging with DDD clinical findings.

Two additional recent studies have examined childhood trauma in people with prominent dpdr; they were not diagnosed with DDD per se. In one study involving a nonclinical sample, participants with clinical levels of de-personalization (about 16% of the total) reported significantly greater emo-tional abuse and neglect than the remaining sample.[13] Furthermore, those with high dpdr had also experienced more adulthood traumatic events, had greater anxiety and emotional overexcitability, and coped worse under stress. The other study examined a young adult community sample and found that childhood emotional maltreatment (abuse and neglect), rather than physical or sexual abuse, accounted for about half of the variability in dpdr severity. Furthermore, dpdr *mediated* the relationship between childhood emotional maltreatment and current psychological distress—it was the link between past experience and present suffering.[14]

There are other kinds of childhood trauma, in addition to the commonly encountered maltreatment, that can figure in the history of those with DDD. Traumatic loss of a loved one during childhood is not uncommon. There are accounts of children or adolescents for whom the death (whether from ill-ness, accident, or suicide) of a parent, sibling, or good friend precipitated chronic dpdr. One patient described a close and loving relationship with his mother. The mother died suddenly and unexpectedly when the boy was 16, and he immediately depersonalized. In the beginning he didn't know what was happening to him and imagined that the strange feeling would go away over time. Indeed, it might initially have reflected the "unreal" aspect of his mourning process. However, the dpdr did not dissipate and became chronic. Another patient had suffered through the slow and terrifying terminal ill-ness of her best high school friend, who eventually died from brain cancer—chronic depersonalization had set in around that time. Yet another DDD patient had lost an older sister to suicide; she harbored a lot of ambivalence toward her lost sister and entered a state of chronic dpdr shortly after the untimely and tragic death.

One study of lifetime traumatic stressors in DDD, *excluding* childhood maltreatment, reported interesting results.[15] Traumatic stressors are defined as stressors outside of the ordinary, and thus more likely to have a lasting psychological impact. The inquiry included 25 major stressors. DDD participants reported significantly more childhood, but not adulthood, traumatic stressors than the healthy comparison group; they also rated these as more stressful and difficult to adjust to. Furthermore, the DDD subgroup with clinically significant childhood maltreatment (about two-thirds, as described earlier) endorsed nearly twice the childhood, as well as adulthood, traumatic stressors than the remaining DDD group. The stressors most frequently reported in DDD, by at least one-third of participants, were as follows (in decreasing order): family member seriously ill or at risk of dying; moving to faraway place or foreign country; and a serious, frightening accident. Taken together, the study's findings suggested that childhood maltreatment is a broader vulnerability in DDD, rendering it more likely that other types of stressors will occur in life, or be experienced as overwhelming and difficult to adapt to should they chance to happen.

Attachment

A person's attachment style, their way of being in relations with others, reflects one's internalized sense of relative security or insecurity surrounding how a close relationship "works." Each person's attachment style is surprisingly stable, from the early years through the course of life. *Secure*, healthy, attachment stems from the basic sense that both oneself and others are "good" and, by extension, that the world and its relationships are reasonably comfortable and safe. Since "secure" people experience themselves and others alike as well-meaning and benevolent, they can comfortably strike a healthy balance between *dependency* (a reasonable expectation that their needs will be understood and taken care of by others) and *autonomy* (a sense that they can competently stand in their own right).

Insecure people are not confident, at heart, that their needs will be met consistently and well enough by others and have adapted accordingly. They struggle with *anxiety* or *avoidance* in their efforts to negotiate the attachment insecurity that close relationships activate. A person with an *anxious-preoccupied* attachment style anxiously clings and depends on others in the hope that they will be taken care of and feel safe—there is over-dependence of the "bad" self on "good" others, and compromised autonomy. A person with a *dismissive* attachment style has a sense of pseudo-autonomy ("good" self) and will readily distance from "bad" others when sensing that their disavowed dependency longings are not being met. Finally, some people have an attachment style known as *fearful*, a mixture of anxiety and avoidance in negotiating relationships. Here, neither *closeness* nor *distance* are stable enough adaptations and solutions for relating to others, so a fear-fully attached person vacillates between the two. Comfort and security are very difficult to experience with this kind of attachment—both closeness and distance breed fear, at its extreme "fear without solution" in the words of re-nowned attachment theorist Mary Main.[16]

Infant research has firmly established that a person's attachment style has been shaped by the second year of life, relatively "hardwired" through the original relationship with the primary caregiver(s). For someone not familiar with attachment theory this may sound stunning—but it's nonetheless true. Though the predominant attachment style can change after the earliest years, it does take a lot for this to occur: new formative experiences with caregivers or other adults, major defining life events, or psychotherapy, to name a few.

Humans do *not* have explicit autobiographical memory for the first couple years of life. No one can tell anyone else what they recall from those years, via the language of our usual memory bank—the hippocampus, the brain center at the core of personal memories, has not yet matured. However, there are other brain systems that are active in the first couple years of life. The amygdala, for example, forms implicit memories, and colors the emotional experience of how relating to others feels—hence the terms "hidden," "rela-tional," or "attachment" trauma, all of which have similar meaning regarding the earliest life experiences. It is trauma that cannot be explicitly recalled and shared, yet its looming presence is reliably inferred in the ways and patterns of relating to others (including psychotherapists—but more about psycho-therapy later).

Attachment trauma has to do with major inconsistencies, unpredicta-bility, misattunement, and communication errors in the early, preverbal, and formative parent–child relationship, creating for the infant/toddler a situa-tion of parental "emotional unavailability." A parent who is not psychologi-cally available enough of the time and in good enough ways is not dyadically relating to the child in a fashion that will promote internalized "felt security."

Though hidden trauma cannot be shared in the typical ways in which later childhood maltreatment usually can be, there is an important and common-sensical connection between attachment trauma and later emotional mal-treatment. Most caregivers typically do not change in major ways as their children grow up, and a child who recalls experiences of emotional abuse or neglect from a young age is more likely to have experienced earlier parental unavailability, and to have struggled with attachment needs.

Attachment is of particular interest in the dissociative disorders, given the intimate connections between trauma and pathological dissociation of all sorts. Dissociative identity disorder (DID) is the quintessential dissociative disorder associated with severe attachment disturbances—often a type of at-tachment known as *disorganized*. Disorganized attachment can be, and has been, observed "with the naked eye," and documented by researchers dating back to Mary Main in 1986; it is an extreme form of fearful attachment. The disorganized toddler behaves in peculiar and disturbing ways when reuniting with the mother after a brief separation, known as the "Strange Situation" in infant research. Instead of the typical behaviors of a secure child, approaching the mother, protesting a bit over the separation, quickly and comfortably settling in, and beginning to play, the disorganized child is at a complete loss—approaches, avoids, looks dazed, freezes, may even col-lapse. The child simply does not know what to do, because there is no safe solution—there is only fear, and confusion.

Unlike the well-known associations of attachment trauma and severe maltreatment with DID, attachment patterns associated with dpdr or DDD have received less attention. An older study, of a university student sample, reported a strong association between depersonalization severity and fearful attachment; in fact, 40% of students with a "depersonalization profile" had a fearful attachment style.[17] Finally, a study published in 2022 used a well-established self-report attachment questionnaire to investigate attachment styles in DDD per se.[18] Of the 42 DDD participants, two-thirds were insecurely attached (compared to one-third of healthy controls), and nearly half (45%) had a fearful attachment style, strikingly higher than the 13% in the comparison group. In other words, fearful attachment was by far the predominant mode of relating in those with the disorder, much more so than anxious-preoccupied or dismissive. Furthermore, fearful attachment was significantly associated with emotional abuse and ne-glect, as well as with physical neglect—the three types of maltreatment most encountered in the disorder. Finally, both fearful attachment and childhood maltreatment predicted the severity of current dissociation, in an additive fashion.

The prevalence of fearful attachment in DDD is consistent with some other features characteristic of the disorder. *Schemas* are enduring structures, at the core of any individual's self-concept, that develop early in life through relationships with primary caregivers. According to Dr. Jeff Young, the developer of schema therapy, there are three overarching schema categories:

Disconnection schemas reflect a sense of defectiveness and emotional inhibition, with themes of relational neglect and deprivation.
Overconnection schemas involve impaired autonomy with themes of dependency and vulnerability.
Exaggerated standards schemas reflect perfectionism and high self-expectations.[19]

In a study using the Schema Questionnaire, both disconnection and overconnection schemas were scored twice as high by the DDD group compared to a healthy control group; exaggerated standards schemas did not differ.[20] These schema findings are consistent with the autonomy and dependency struggles that are inherent to a fearful attachment style.

Temperament is another aspect of DDD consistent with the prevalence of fearful attachment. Every child is born with a particular temperament, an innate biological disposition in how they experience the world and regulate emotions, adversity or its absence aside (we already discussed how an innate propensity for normative dissociation is another sort of trait in DDD). Temperament is a trait and, like attachment style, carries great stability over the life span, constituting one building block for later adult personality. We give just one example here of a major temperament study, possibly relevant to DDD. This prospective study was carried out over 30 years (a very long time for any research project) and was published in 2020 in the *Proceedings of the National Academy of Sciences*.[21] It reported that infants rated high on the temperament of *behavioral inhibition* (cautious and fearful in unfamiliar situations) were more likely by the time they reached adulthood, at the age of 26, to have a certain kind of personality low on extraversion and high on neuroticism (low positive emotion, proneness to anxiety and depression).

When one does not have the luxury of measuring temperament at birth and tracking it to adulthood, an adequate approximation of temperament can be obtained by a validated adulthood questionnaire that measures temperament. Dr. Robert Cloninger is a well-known researcher of temperament and personality, and he originally proposed three temperament dimensions: *novelty-seeking, reward-dependence,* and *harm-avoidance.* The U.S. group used this Tridimensional Personality Questionnaire to investigate temperament in DDD.[20] Though the DDD group did not differ in novelty-seeking or in reward-dependence from the healthy comparison group, harm-avoidance was rated almost twice as high—furthermore, the greater the harm avoidance, the stronger the dissociation severity. When this finding of harm-avoidant temperament is thought about alongside a fearful attachment style, an interesting possibility arises. It could it be those individuals born with a behaviorally inhibited and harm-avoidant temperament, as well as with an innate propensity to dissociate, are more likely, if exposed to significant childhood adversity, to develop a fearful attachment style and pathological dissociative symptoms. Little by little, pieces of the DDD puzzle fall into place.

No Words for Emotions

People who feel secure are generally more able to know and to handle their emotions, a process referred to as *emotional processing.* Feelings are of central importance and value to healthy human adaptation and survival, and to wellbeing. When a person does not know what they are feeling, or how to make sense of what they are feeling, they are at a great disadvantage in assessing their inner world, their relationships, and all the situations they encounter in life. Emotional processing occurs both consciously and unconsciously but, generally speaking, the more precarious or difficult the situation one finds oneself in, the greater the need for conscious processing to prevent states of overwhelmingness and psychic collapse. However, dissociation, as a state of "knowing and not knowing," is tricky in this respect. Can a person, child or adult, afford to know their emotional states if these are too unsafe, too dangerous? And here enters alexithymia.

Alexithymia, aptly coined from the Greek "no words for emotions," means just that. It is a relative deficit in the self-awareness of emotions, which inherently leads to difficulty processing and regulating emotions and to an emotionally constricted way of being. Both one's own emotional world and that of others are less accessible to a person with alexithymia. In relationships, and in talk therapy, people with alexithymia have trouble talking about their feelings, as well as comprehending the feelings of others and being empathic. Alexithymia can be reliably quantified and measured, and the Toronto Alexithymia Scale (TAS) is one of the most widely used questionnaires to this purpose.[22]

The TAS measures three aspects of alexithymia: *difficulty identifying feelings, difficulty describing feelings,* and *externally oriented thinking.* Any person's alexithymia can have *primary* and *secondary* components. Primary alexithymia is a lifelong characteristic, a trait, in part genetically influenced and in part shaped at the very start of life in the context of negative experiences with primary caregivers and attachment disturbances. Secondary alexithymia occurs later, as a state rather than a trait, in response to sociocultural expectations as well as personal life experiences. Though not cut-and-dried, difficulty identifying feelings is believed to be more primary, whereas difficulty expressing feelings is more secondary.

Clinically meaningful "high" alexithymia in the general population is thought to occur in about one out of 10 people, defined as a total score of 61 or higher on the TAS. Alexithymia has been studied in DDD, and the findings are not surprising: both the U.S. and the U.K. groups have confirmed the presence of marked alexithymia in the disorder. The New York group reported that 23% of those with DDD had "difficulty identifying feelings" and 33% had "difficulty describing feelings," at clinically relevant levels that used established TAS subscale cutoff scores. The "difficulty identifying feelings" score, in and of itself, predicted whether a study participant belonged to the DDD or the healthy control group with a 78% accuracy. Furthermore, this same score was strongly associated with dpdr severity.[23] For "total" alexithymia, of 40 DDD participants studied by the group 25% scored high and 20% scored moderate; simply put, nearly half of DDD patients were characterized by elevated alexithymia.

A neuroimaging study of nine DDD patients reported on by the London group replicated similar findings: two had high alexithymia, four moderate, and three low[24] (this study mapped out the different facets of alexithymia onto different brain regions—but more about this in the next chapter).

As already discussed, knowing what one feels and being able to put it into words are key to emotional processing and regulation, allowing a person to be mindful (aware of their inner experience) and to mentalize (reflect and make meaning). Mindlessness is, in effect, a relative absence of mindfulness and mentalization. In a sample of medical students, the German group found that childhood emotional maltreatment was positively associated with depersonalization severity and negatively associated with mindfulness.[25] In other words, those who had experienced emotional trauma when growing up understandably had more trouble being aware of their emotional states, and this is turn fueled a depersonalized way of being. Though mentalization per se has not yet been studied in DDD, we can be almost certain that it is impaired, at least in those who have higher alexithymia and lower mindfulness. If a person has trouble knowing and describing what they feel, and trouble being attentive to their emotional state, they most certainly will have difficulty reflecting on and making sense of their own emotional world, and that of others. The many pieces of the DDD puzzle continue to fall into place.

Cognition

Cognitive complaints are common in DDD. Patients often tell that their attention and memory has changed; it's not like before. Subjectively they may have trouble pinpointing if the problem is more with inattentiveness or with memory (if any stimulus is not attended to in the first place, it is less likely to be remembered). The complaints apply not only to work but also to simple day-to-day tasks, as well as to interactions with others and partaking in conversations. For a fraction of DDD patients, cognitive difficulties can be the most troubling symptom of the disorder, and quite debilitating. Adding to this picture, for some with DDD, the incessant preoccupation over their state of mind and its implications further fuels the distraction and inattentiveness. In fact, even those with DDD who are able to hold on to more demanding jobs often report that they are not performing at their full capacity; their ability to attend to information and to process it feels very impaired. So, the story of cognition in DDD is an important one to investigate and better understand.

The New York research group has conducted several cognition studies in DDD. These serial studies methodically replicated earlier findings, narrowed in on cognitive domains of interest in the disorder, and explored the impact of emotions on attention and memory. Cognitive studies use batteries of established, widely used cognitive tests to objectively measure "performance" in all the major domains of human cognition and to hone in on areas of particular interest; some tests are pencil-and-paper, others are computerized. The cognitive findings in DDD paint a rather consistent picture, one of generally intact cognitive functioning, with some pockets of difficulty, and particular ways of cognitively processing emotional material.

The first study of cognition in 15 DDD participants reported that general intelligence, working memory, and executive functioning were all intact, and did not differ from the healthy control group.[26] The study also found that once information had been processed and encoded successfully, there appeared to be no problem retaining and using it; long-term memory was intact (this important finding of overall intact general cognition in DDD was confirmed by two subsequent studies[27,28]). However, the study identified some difficulties with "early information processing" having to do with the effortful control of perception and attention, consequently leading to diminished short-term memory, verbal and visual. This finding of diminished visual and verbal immediate recall was replicated in a subsequent study,[27] and it was concluded that DDD "is associated with cognitive disruptions in early perceptual and attentional processes" (p. 983).

It became apparent that there was a need to take a closer look at, and to dissect, all the complex components of *attention*. One key finding, later replicated, was that *selective* attention is intact in DDD.[26,28] Selective attention was measured by what is known as the Stroop Task, a classic test of cognition developed in 1935 by American psychologist John Stroop (and readily available online on various brain game websites for those who may be curious). When taking this test, a person must declare, as fast as possible, the *color* in which a word is printed while ignoring any *interference* that the word itself may pose (e.g., if the word "blue" is printed in green, test-takers must respond "green"). Another DDD study again demonstrated that selective attention is intact in DDD, using a different test called the Digit Span with Distracters. However, this study also found an inverse relationship between dissociation severity and test performance—in other words, the more depersonalized a person with DDD was, the harder it became to stay selectively focused.[27]

Another type of attention is known as *sustained* attention, and it reflects how well a person can stay on target during a prolonged attentional task, and not be distracted by a variety of extraneous stimuli that are presented during testing (attention deficit disorder is the hallmark condition in which this function is compromised). Sustained attention is measured by the, not surprisingly named, Continuous Performance test. Again, the DDD group was found to perform overall fine on this test, yet *not* so for its highest level of difficulty: in the presence of "high-demand distracters," sustaining attention was compromised by distraction.[26]

Divided attention is yet another important attentional capacity, and was studied next in DDD.[28] Here, participants were presented with a challenging task that requires dividing attention between two conflicting sets of stimuli. A Modified Stroop Task was used to test this function, during which a person must read out colors as fast as possible (as described earlier) while at the same time *remembering* the words printed in color (rather than simply *ignoring* them as in the standard selective-attention Stroop Task). DDD participants had no problem effectively dividing their attention, just like the healthy controls. However, they did this in a *preferential* manner that speaks to the early information processing of *emotional* material in the disorder.

In the Modified Stroop Task, some words were neutral while others were "emotional" (dissociation and trauma related), and the study findings were quite interesting.[28] DDD patients favored lesser interference by words and color-named faster than healthy controls, but at the expense of subsequently recalling the words. Simply put, they demonstrated a cognitive preference for pre-semantic, sensory (visual) early information processing.

What could such a cognitive style possibly translate into in real life? Imagine the young child of a caregiver who yells and screams, feeling frightened, demeaned, and wanting to shut it all out if they could. In this scenario, the child could attend to the actual words uttered by the caregiver or, if they have a dissociative propensity toward dividing attention, the child could instead hone in on the color of the adult's clothing, or the wallpaper in the background of the room. The latter strategy carries emotional gain, for the moment at least. Highly disturbing semantic information (verbal abuse) can be filtered out some and remembered less, while the safer (emotionally irrelevant) colors of the surrounding environment are being preferentially attended to. The investigators concluded there this was evidence for "emotionally avoidant information processing" in the disorder.

Yet another finding in this study provided further support for emotionally avoidant information processing in DDD. The investigators conducted a memory test for neutral versus negative words that was administered twice, once before and again after a standardized psychological stressor known as the Trier Social Stress Test. The DDD group demonstrated significantly better recall for neutral versus negative words pre-stress and for negative versus neutral words post-stress, whereas the healthy group demonstrated the exact opposite pattern.[28] This finding tells us that the baseline dissociative capacity to "ignore" negative information broke down under stress, and the negative information then prevailed. Though this is a commonsensically understandable cognitive strategy in people with histories of trauma (not remembering the negative), it is less useful as a general life adaptation. It is easier to process emotionally disturbing material when in a relatively quiescent state of mind, as the healthy control group did, than in a stressed state of mind when the disturbing material finally "breaks through." The key finding of emotionally avoidant information processing in DDD is consistent with the emotional maltreatment, relational fear, alexithymia, and diminished mindfulness that we have already laid out in this chapter.

In conclusion, the cognition findings encountered in DDD are for the most part subtle: general cognitive abilities are intact, but there is some difficulty with early attentional and perceptual processing, and a cognitive bias away from emotional information. Yet patients may very much complain of cognitive struggles, which to them feel very real, and which can interfere with daily cognitive performance, as well as vivid emotional recollection of past experience. The objective cognitive findings obtained thus far in DDD can help explain the difficulty attending to demanding work and the vulnerability to distraction, as well as the blunting that comes with avoiding emotional material. There is probably a subjective component to how DDD patients experience their own cognitive processes as well (commonly referred to as metacognition). It could well be that feeling unreal, spaced, and detached colors one's own perception of one's cognitive capacities in negative ways, worse than actual performance demonstrates or suggests. The "unreal" perception of one's own cognition must take a toll, leaving some with DDD feeling more cognitively impaired than they "really" are.

A Fear-Based Trauma Model for the Genesis of DDD

It is probably fair to say that leading investigators of DDD do not weigh in on the four areas discussed in this chapter (trauma, attachment, alexithymia, cognition) in quite the same way. The British group leans more heavily toward an anxiety model of the disorder. The U.S. group leans more heavily toward a trauma model. The German group seems to weigh in halfway. Let us consider an integration of the DDD findings in this chapter: trait dissociative propensity, emotional maltreatment, fearful attachment, overconnection and disconnection schemas, harm-avoidant temperament, alexithymia, diminished mindfulness, and impaired early informational and emotional processing—with dpdr as the outcome. An anxiety-based model puts greater emphasis on personal and familial anxiety predispositions and on stressful anxiety-provoking events, precipitating the vicious cycle of worry, ruminations, and self-perpetuating symptoms characteristic of anxiety conditions. A trauma-based model places emphasis on the fearful adaptation to emotional maltreatment and attachment trauma, and to the concomitant contributions of alexithymia and emotionally avoidant processing, all together precipitating a dissociative, unreal, and emotionally impoverished way of experiencing the self and being in the world.

Fear and anxiety are not the same. Fear is an emotional reaction to specific psychological dangers in the present, even if more "real" in early life and more "triggered" in the now. Anxiety is not a basic emotion; it is a diffuse, contentless (though it will vicariously latch on to contents) signal centered on the possibility of future harm; it resides in what will come more than in the now. Both models accommodate both a dissociative diathesis and an anxiety-proneness. However, dpdr likely requires more than anxiety-proneness coupled with elevated normative dissociation and some degree of alexithymia to happen. These pieces may be necessary but not sufficient. It is the pervasive emotional trauma and fear-centered relating that tips an anxiety- and dissociation- prone individual into one with the dissociative disorder of DDD.

DDD Clinical Profile, Part II

- Emotional maltreatment (abuse and neglect) is common.
- Fearful attachment style predominates.
- Relationship schemas involve themes of overconnection and underconnection, reflecting compromised autonomy and dependency.
- Anxious temperament (behavioral inhibition) may contribute to fearful attachment in the face of early adversity.
- Alexithymia is common and contributes to difficulties with emotional processing and with mindfulness/mentalization.

- Most major cognitive domains are intact.
- Delineated cognitive difficulties involve a vulnerability to attentional overload under high distraction, a bias for perceptual over semantic information, and an emotionally avoidant cognitive style.

Part I of the DDD Clinical Profile was in Chapter 6.

8

Neurobiology

The human brain has 100 billion neurons, each neuron connected to 10 thousand other neurons. Sitting on your shoulders is the most complicated object in the known universe.

—Michio Kaku

Despite Kaku's astute observation, popular culture has developed a tendency to liken the brain to a computer or explain serious disorders in terms of simple chemical imbalances. Such generalizations just don't do this fascinating organ justice. Let's first take a scientific look at the basic anatomy and function of the brain, then move on to a closer look at what is known about the brain in depersonalization/derealization disorder (DDD).

Any scientific hypothesis, no matter how strong it seems in theory, needs empirical testing. Data need to be collected in the real world. As Thomas Kuhn observed, we can never *prove* a scientific model with certainty—better-fitting or more comprehensive models could arise at any future time. We can, however, *disprove* a scientific model, by collecting empirical information, data, in the real world that is simply not compatible with the model. What then is the actual evidence for the various biological models of DDD?

The Doors of Perception: Sensory Association Cortex and Sensory Unreality

The most recently evolved part of the human brain is the neocortex, which lies on the surface, enveloping and connecting to the deeper, older structures within. One part of the cortex is the sensory cortex, which is responsible for receiving sensory information encoded by our various sensory organs, and deciphering and translating it into known perceptual entities, "percepts," that we can make sense of. This information is transmitted and processed

Feeling Unreal. Second Edition. Daphne Simeon and Jeffrey Abugel, Oxford University Press. © Oxford University Press 2023. DOI: 10.1093/oso/9780197622445.003.0008

via a network of interacting brain cells called neurons. These communicate with each other via the various substances that together are known as neurotransmitters.

When we perceive something, say a hand being extended to us for a handshake, our brain makes sense of it as a known entity that belongs to the "hand" category—it is experienced as something quite familiar, with numerous perceptual associations, and it may even spark various emotional and autobiographical memories. Sensory input, such as visual (sight), auditory (hearing), olfactory (smell), gustatory (taste), or somatosensory (touch, pain, position, movement), is first processed in the simplest sensory areas of the cortex known as the primary sensory cortex. The primary cortex for visual input sits in the occipital lobe of the brain. For sound and smell it's located in parts of the temporal lobe. And for somatic sensations it is in the parietal lobe (see Figure 8.1). These areas receive the sensory information and then relay it to more complex sensory cortical areas that synthesize perceptual information within each separate sensory modality. These more complex regions are known as the secondary unimodal association areas. In our example of the human hand, the visual appearance of the newly perceived object is matched against a preexisting template of a hand stored in the visual association area of the cortex. There it's perceived as something known.

Next, all these individual (unimodal) sensory aspects of the hand come together to form the complex and unique "experience" of a hand in what are known as the cross-modal or polymodal sensory association areas of

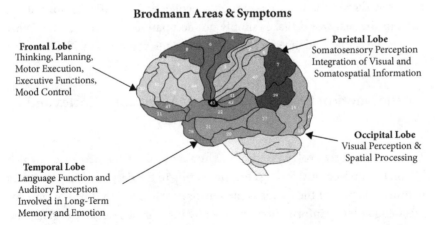

Figure 8.1 Brodmann areas of the human cortex and their associated major functions. (Source: Big8/Shutterstock.)

the brain. Similarly, other attributes of the hand are matched against other sensory templates. Any possible scent of the hand is matched against an olfactory sensory template; any sound it might make is matched against an auditory sensory template. There is a gustatory template for the possible tastes associated with a hand, and the feeling of holding hands, shaking hands, or being struck by a hand in anger has a somatosensory template. These areas are crucial perceptual areas responsible for the higher-level integration of all sensory input across the various sensory modalities. One such area is known as the *inferior parietal lobule* or *temporoparietal junction* (TPJ), a portion of the parietal lobe consisting of the supramarginal and angular gyrus, strategically seated right at the junction of the parietal lobe with the temporal and occipital lobes (see Figure 8.1). The TPJ is critical to our ability to have a well-integrated body schema—that is, an intact and unified physical sense of self. Does depersonalization come to mind here? Clearly it does.

In fact, the entire neurological literature, when reviewed very carefully from the viewpoint of one well versed in psychiatric syndromes, can be very revealing. Structural abnormalities of the brain, such as those that can result from head injury, stroke, epilepsy, tumors, and innumerable other conditions, can "mimic" just about anything "psychiatric": psychosis, depression, mania, anxiety, and so on. Dissociation and depersonalization are no exception. A careful reading of the neurological literature does suggest a unique role for portions of the posterior sensory cortex (temporal, parietal, and occipital) in mediating depersonalization-like experiences. Let's take a look then at reports of depersonalization in the neurological literature.

When something is amiss in the TPJ, a person's core sense of the "body self" can be affected. Certain neurological syndromes, known as "neglect syndromes" or asomatognosia, result from strokes in the right TPJ and are reminiscent of the disembodiment of depersonalization. The afflicted person with such a stroke ignores the left side of the body, as if it does not exist; though there is no motor weakness, the left arm or leg may fall into disuse.[1] There is a soft analogy to depersonalization here—even though people with depersonalization know intellectually that their body exists, they don't feel the relation to their body in a normal way, so it's experienced *as if* it does not exist. In fact, back in 1954 the British physician Ackner reported that tumors in the inferior parietal cortex can manifest with frank depersonalization.[2] Neurological problems in the parietal lobes other than strokes can also produce symptoms akin to depersonalization. Depersonalization experiences have also been described in seizures generating in the parietal lobes; these can present with symptoms like somatosensory auras, disturbances of body image, vertiginous sensations, and visual illusions.[3] And a report in the prestigious journal *Nature* described a patient with refractory parietal lobe epilepsy who underwent a direct brain stimulation procedure to better map the damaged section of her brain. Various areas of the brain were electrically stimulated, but when the right TPJ was probed the patient experienced, for the first time, repeated out-of-body sensations.[4]

The neurologist Wilder G. Penfield is renowned for his decades of seminal work in epilepsy, conducted in the 1940s through the 1960s at McGill University in Montreal, one of the oldest and most renowned medical schools in the new world. Dr. Penfield helped elucidate many of the structures and functions of the brain, largely through his efforts to understand, map, and surgically treat epilepsy, in particular temporal lobe epilepsy (TLE). Penfield proposed what is referred to as the "temporal lobe hypothesis" of depersonalization in 1950. He wrote about "clear sensations of not being present or floating away . . . far off and out of this world," which were produced by electrical stimulation of specific areas of the temporal cortex, the superior temporal gyrus, and the middle temporal gyrus.[5] In trying to understand his patients' clear and vivid experiences of pure depersonalization, Penfield postulated that what was occurring was an alteration in the usual mechanisms of comparing immediate sensory perceptions against existing memory records in the brain that gave these percepts emotional coloring and relevance. This gets to the core of the depersonalization experience because it has to do with the subjective sense of *unfamiliarity*. Perceptions *both* of the self and of the things around us that should feel familiar, and therefore real, do not feel familiar and real in depersonalization/derealization (dpdr), because they are not appropriately emotionally tagged as *known* against preexisting memory records. Penfield's "temporal lobe hypothesis" is supported by the frequent occurrence of depersonalization in patients with TLE: patients who have seizures generating in the left temporal lobe often experience dpdr.[6]

Yet another set of pertinent studies in healthy volunteers has attempted to examine what happens in the brain when we look at stimuli that are experienced as familiar or unfamiliar; it is needless to say how relevant this might be to depersonalization, where the familiar is experienced as unfamiliar. These studies of visual familiarity found that unfamiliar faces narrowly activated only unimodal visual association areas, whereas familiar (or famous) faces produced more widespread activation of transmodal association areas, specifically the middle temporal gyrus (see TLE) and the angular gyrus (TPJ).[7] These findings again might imply that in depersonalization there is a failure of sensory association cortex integration, especially at the level of higher associations and connections responsible for registering the familiar as such.

Dr. Simeon's group was the first to demonstrate that the unreality experiences of DDD may be associated with widespread dysfunction of the sensory association cortex—all the neurological findings just presented are in sync with such a hypothesis.[8] A positron emission tomography (PET) imaging study was published in the *American Journal of Psychiatry* in 2000, comparing people with DDD to a healthy control group. All participants took a standardized verbal memory test to control for mental activity during the uptake of the radioactive glucose by the brain (the two groups performed similarly on this test). All the DDD participants were suffering from continuous dpdr, including at the timepoint when they were scanned. The findings were quite telling. There was no difference in brain activity between the two groups for the entire anterior portion of the brain, including the frontal and the cingulate cortex (these are the areas responsible for many higher cognitive functions such as planning and executing our daily tasks, emotional experiencing and regulation, and experiences of selfhood). All the differences in activity found between the two groups were localized in the *posterior cortex* (temporal, parietal, and occipital).

A closer look at very specific brain areas, known as Brodmann areas (BA; Figure 8.1), revealed that the two groups differed in occipital BA 19, temporal BA 21 and 22, and parietal BA 7B and 39.[8] Importantly, all these areas are parts of the "sensory association cortex," responsible for processing sensory stimuli within each sensory modality, as well as making the various associations across different sensory modalities. BA 19 is part of the secondary visual cortex, crucial to processing many aspects of vision, including light intensity as well as depth perception. DDD patients often report anomalies in these sensory experiences. BA 21 and 22 are auditory association areas that sit in the temporal lobe. They are associated with both visual and auditory processing, of nonverbal complex sounds (right side) as well as language processing (left side).

Regarding the parietal regions differing in brain activity between the two groups, BA 7B is the region involved in secondary somatosensory processing, and has complex connections with visual, proprioceptive (internal bodily stimuli), auditory, and vestibular (balance-related) brain areas. The region is also implicated in pain perception, as well as in early attentional processes, as part of the frontoparietal attentional network. Importantly, there was a strong relationship between greater depersonalization severity and higher activity in this BA. BA 39, also known as the angular gyrus, is part of the TPJ, as we already discussed (in Chapter 10 we will see that this region is now an established target for DDD repetitive transcranial magnetic stimulation [TMS] treatment).

The TPJ functions as a parieto-temporo-occipital crossroad of sorts—it subsumes cross-modal connectivity, is crucial to a well-integrated body schema, and has extensive projections to the prefrontal cortex as well as to the limbic system. Adding to its many functions, the TPJ has also emerged as a key region for emotional processing. As mentioned earlier, it is involved in the discrimination of familiar from unfamiliar faces.[8] The TPJ is also involved in lower-level attentional social processing, via the so-called ventral attention network. Neuroscientists Adolphs and Damasio, in a paper published in the *Journal of Neuroscience* in 2000, reported that neurological patients with lesions in the TPJ had trouble accurately rating the intensity of basic emotions expressed by faces, across the whole range of emotions spanning happiness, surprise, fear, anger, disgust, and sadness.[9] Damage to the left TPJ impeded patients' ability to accurately *name* the emotions of facial expressions, whereas damage to the *right* TPJ lessened the patients' ability to accurately sort emotions into categories. These findings immediately bring to mind the alexithymia encountered in many DDD patients (see Chapter 7). By now it's apparent then that the perceptions of bodily states and emotional states are intimately related, and parietal regions are central to these functions.

In summary, then, the DDD PET imaging study was the first to show that widespread changes in sensory cortical activity are salient to DDD, consistent with a long lineage of neurological findings. A few years later, in 2005, a study was published in the *Journal of Neuroscience* directly linking the TPJ to transient out-of-body experiences (OBEs) in healthy volunteers.[10] Using evoked potential mapping, the investigators found that the TPJ was selectively activated when the volunteers were asked to imagine themselves in the position and visual perspective like that of someone experiencing a spontaneous OBE. They also found that interference with TPJ functioning by TMS blocked the participants' capacity to mentally transform their normal body experience into an OBE. This TPJ function was specific to one's own body and had nothing to do with imagined spatial transformations of external objects. The investigators concluded, as had already been shown in DDD, that the TPJ is "a crucial structure for the conscious experience of the normal self, mediating spatial unity of self and body" (p. 550).

Though this far we've focused on individual cortical areas with altered activity in DDD, there is a bigger picture of what is known as brain *connectivity*, having to do with the ways different areas communicate with each other in the usual ways, or in disrupted ways generally referred to as brain "dysconnectivity." The major neurotransmitters that regulate corticocortical connectivity are the excitatory neurotransmitter glutamate and the inhibitory neurotransmitter GABA. Back in 1998, Dr. John Krystal and colleagues, from Yale University, proposed a "corticocortical dysconnectivity" model for dissociation, centering on the glutamate system.[11] The evidence primarily came from people with posttraumatic stress disorder (PTSD), but was relevant to the mechanisms of dissociation. It was further proposed that "thalamo-cortical dysconnectivity" also needs be considered in dissociation. The thalamus is a critical brain region that serves as an entry gate for the processing of sensations coming in from our various sensory organs, then relaying the information to various parts of the cortex (see later in this chapter for more on the thalamus).

Corticocortical connectivity is facilitated by what's known as the NMDA (*N*-methyl-D-aspartate) receptor, the receptor for the excitatory neurotransmitter glutamate. When people are given ketamine, an NMDA receptor blocker also known as a "dissociative anesthetic" (or "Special K" in street jargon), they fall into deep dissociative states (more on ketamine in dissociation later). In the occasional individual, DDD is initially triggered by the casual use of ketamine (see Chapter 6). And we will later see that lamotrigine, a medication helpful in treating DDD, may work by impacting glutamate transmission (see Chapter 10). Furthermore, there might even be a chemical link here to a much more common DDD-triggering drug, marijuana—in addition to their action on the brain's endogenous cannabinoid receptors, cannabinoids are known to inhibit glutamate release.

Known and Unknown Memories: Amygdala and Hippocampus

Now back to the extended hand. Perceiving this familiar part of a person evokes not only the known percept of a hand, but possibly all kinds of associated thoughts, feelings, and memories. The sensory association areas of the cortex have connections to the prefrontal cortex, which allows us to have thoughts about the hand, to the frontal motor cortex involved in executing an appropriate action in response to the handshake, and to the limbic cortex involved in evoking emotional memories surrounding the particular handshake.

Neuroscience research has determined that the initial formation of emotional memories is contingent on the activation of two tiny, almond-size bilateral brain structures known as the *amygdala* (from the Greek root word for almond), embedded deep in the temporal lobes. The amygdala belongs to the limbic system (see Figure 8.2), an ancestral part of the brain that has not changed much over the course of evolution from the reptiles to *Homo sapiens*. The amygdala plays a central role in a variety of instinctually driven emotional processes such as the conditioned fear response (e.g., when a laboratory animal responds negatively to a light or sound because it has been consistently paired to a mild electric shock in the past), the automatic reading of emotional facial expressions, as well as the formation of implicit emotional memories. Much has been researched and written about the amygdala as the seat of a central animal emotion—*fear*. Not surprisingly, many imaging studies have found that that the amygdala is hyperresponsive to potential threat in PTSD.[12] Conversely, one might speculate that in dissociative states characterized by hypoemotionality, the amygdala would be hyporeactive when a person is emotionally stimulated.

Equally important within our limbic system is the *hippocampus*. The hippocampus is the seat of our autobiographical memories—that is, all the explicit (conscious) memories that make up the story of our lives, stored

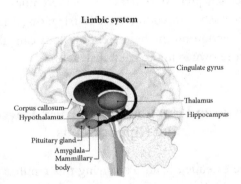

Figure 8.2 Diagram of the limbic system. (Source: Designua/Shutterstock.)

contextually with the "stamp" of time, place, and details of what occurred. The encoding, storage, and retrieval of our personal memories is a highly complex process involving the hippocampus as well as other extended cortical networks. An autobiographical memory cannot be "retrieved" if an early "kernel" of the memory is not activated in the hippocampus, which serves as the epicenter of the distributed memory network in the brain. Of course, no autobiographical memory could be retrieved if it was not encoded in the first place. Emotional memory difficulties associated with depersonalization appear to be more related to early information processing and *initial* memory encoding (see the section on cognition in the previous chapter), distinguishing it from dissociative conditions like amnesia, where the problem lies with the compartmentalization of encoded memories and with their retrieval.

The amygdala and hippocampus are two very important subcortical structures in the brain. The amygdala is crucial to the initial (subcortical) processing of fear and other emotions before these are processed at a higher cortical level, and it is the seat of emotional memory. It's the source of the organism's *immediate* fight-or-flight response, whereas the hippocampus's purpose lies in the consolidation of information, and the retaining of autobiographical and episodic memories—personal contextualized stories of what we have experienced. These two brain structures can operate quite independently of each other—which raises a very interesting possibility. A person may have *little or no* memory of something that happened to them, especially something traumatic, because a clear autobiographical memory of the event may not have been registered by the hippocampus under great stress. But on the other hand, there may be a different kind of record of the event mediated by the amygdala—of the associated *feelings* that the experience involved. If at some future time, a person encounters something reminiscent of an old trauma, they may have an intense emotional and behavioral reaction based what the amygdala "know," but no concrete memory for what it was.

The renowned neuroscientist Joseph LeDoux described the implications of this distinction between explicit and implicit memory in his widely read book *The Emotional Brain* (1996).[13] LeDoux explains that the knowledge that a particular incident was terrifying is a declarative memory about an emotional experience, mediated by the hippocampus and its connections. On the other hand, the intense emotional response evoked during the event (and during its later recollection) activates the implicit memory system and involves the amygdala and its connections. Under sufficiently intense or prolonged stress, there can occur a stress hormone (cortisol)-mediated shutdown of the hippocampus, leading to impaired functioning of the explicit and conscious memory system. At the same time, the stress does not interfere with, and may even enhance, amygdala functioning. According to LeDoux, a person may have poor explicit (conscious), yet powerful implicit (unconscious) emotional memory for a traumatic event.[13] This distinction is crucially relevant to understanding dissociative and other traumatic phenomena. Stimuli may activate the amygdala without activating conscious memories, eliciting an intense emotional state that the individual has no formulated understanding of, "knows and does not know."

There is another crucial difference between the implicit and explicit memory systems, which is a developmental one (see the section on attachment in the previous chapter). It accounts for why early life traumas, before the age of two or so, can be implicitly known but not explicitly remembered. While the amygdala is fully developed at birth, the hippocampus takes over two years to mature. The consequence is what Freud first labeled as "infantile amnesia:" he was correct about the observation that children have no conscious memories from the first two or three years of life, but incorrect in his attribution. The cause is not psychological repression of early memories, but rather a neurodevelopmental constraint founded on the differential maturation of the two organs. This basic and straightforward neurobiological fact is highly explanatory when it comes to very early life adversity. Our patients cannot tell us about it with words because they do not explicitly recall it. But they can behave in ways, "reenactments" as these are commonly referred to, that may suggest the presence of such early traumas. Aptly, infant researcher Lyons-Ruth coined the term "hidden traumas of infancy" for such phenomena. The sections that follow demonstrate that the hippocampus *has not* been implicated in DDD—likely not surprising given the general intactness of autobiographical memory—while the amygdala and other structures involved in emotional processing and memory, such as the insula, *have* been implicated.

Insula: The Island of Emotion

The insula is a region seated deep inside the brain where the frontal, temporal, and parietal lobes meet. The label "hidden fifth lobe" hints at its uniquely important functions in the human brain: it is a "hub linking large-scale brain systems" (R581).[14] The insula is associated with interoceptive (internal sensation) awareness, in close communication with the parietal cortex, registering bodily sensations, temperature, and pain. It also receives sensory information from the environment, and plays an important role in the integration of various sensory modalities such as vision, smell, and taste. It then links sensory input to emotion—for example, an aversive sight, or smell, or taste will elicit the primal emotion of disgust (more about this follows). As a hub for both sensory and emotional processing, and their integration, the insula monitors bodily and emotional inner states, as well as the external environment, and determines the valence (positive or negative) of internal and external stimuli, thus generating a "prediction" of how to best react. Given all these functions, the insula is yet another brain area of potential interest in DDD—one would predict insular hyporeactivity in response to provoking stimuli, given the sensory and emotional blunting often associated with dpdr.

Cortico-Limbic Disconnection and Hypoemotionality

In 1998, a neurobiological model of depersonalization known as "cortico-limbic disconnection" was put forth by Mauricio Sierra and German Berrios, from the Cambridge Department of Psychiatry.[15] It proposed that depersonalization involves a dysconnectivity between certain parts of the brain that are not functioning in sync: hyperactivation of the prefrontal cortex, responsible for the cognitive processing and downregulation of our emotional experiences, is overly inhibiting the limbic system, which mediates the more emotional aspects of our experiences. This reciprocal prefrontal activation and limbic inhibition subsumes the hypoemotionality encountered in DDD.

There is research evidence supporting this model. Cannabinoids, such as marijuana, are well known to induce transient depersonalization in many during the "high," and even trigger prolonged dpdr in those with presumed underlying vulnerability (see Chapter 6). Depersonalization-type symptoms have been induced in healthy people through chemical means and then visualized by brain imagery. One PET study reported that administration of tetrahydrocannabinol (THC; marijuana) to healthy volunteers resulted in increased brain activity in the prefrontal and anterior cingulate cortex (the latter modulates attention); this increase correlated with the severity of THC-induced depersonalization.[16] At the same time, the volunteers experienced a decrease in subcortical activity in limbic areas. These findings supported the "cortico-limbic" disconnection hypothesis just described: *hyper*-active prefrontal and *hypo*-active limbic system.

In 2001, researchers from the London Institute of Psychiatry published their first neuroimaging study lending direct support to this brain model in DDD, aptly titled "Thinking Without Feeling."[17] They compared depersonalized patients, patients with obsessive-compulsive disorder (OCD), and healthy volunteers. Researchers used the functional magnetic resonance imaging (fMRI) technique, which detects changes in activity in different parts of the brain in real moment-to-moment sequential timeframes, as people are presented with different tasks. All participants were shown picture sets of neutral and aversive (disgusting) objects—a cockroach was depicted in one set, for instance, as well as open wounds in another. Disgust is a primal emotion, one of the six core emotions that psychologist Paul Ekman defined as universal and cross-cultural (the others are fear, sadness, joy, anger, and surprise).[18]

The findings revealed that contrary to healthy and OCD individuals, depersonalized patients showed a heightened activation in their prefrontal cortex but did *not* activate the insula, the limbic area responsible for experiencing the primal emotion of disgust, in response to the aversive pictures. Participants also rated the pictures for emotional content: though DDD participants intellectually knew which stimuli were disgusting, their emotional experience was less aversive than that of the other two groups .

Over the past two decades, the Institute of Psychiatry in London has conducted a series of fMRI studies that have generally affirmed the attenuation of emotional responses in DDD, subsumed by various kinds of cortico-limbic miscommunications. Here we present some selected studies of interest. One fMRI study, by Dr. Lemche and colleagues, found attenuated responses to both happy and sad emotions in the disorder.[19] Whereas the healthy control group showed increasing limbic activation in response to increasing stimulus emotional intensity, the DDD group showed decreasing limbic activation to increasing emotion—in the amygdala for sadness and in the hypothalamus for happiness. And, there was the expected concomitant hyperactivation of the posterior prefrontal cortex, inhibiting limbic reactivity.

An fMRI study by Dr. Medford and colleagues had encouraging treatment implications.[20] It found that before treatment, the insula of DDD participants had reduced emotional reactivity. After treatment with the medication lamotrigine, those DDD patients whose symptoms improved showed increased insula reactivity to both happy and sad expressions. Additionally, the ventrolateral prefrontal cortex was directly implicated in the "top-down" inhibition of the insula.

Another fMRI study, also by Dr. Medford and colleagues, examined emotional memory in DDD.[21] Compared to healthy controls, DDD patients did not show the expected enhancement of memory for neutral words embedded in an emotional context. They also showed no activation of the brain's emotional processing areas, neither during the encoding nor the recognition of emotional material. The study contributed to the growing evidence of diminished processing of emotionally salient information in the disorder.

Yet another fMRI study by Dr. Lemche and colleagues examined the neurobiology of alexithymia.[22] We discussed alexithymia in the previous chapter, how common it is in DDD, and how it contributes to the hypoemotionality often present in those with the condition. The nine DDD participants in this study had varying degrees of alexithymia, ranging from high to moderate to low (again, see Chapter 7), and as usual were compared to healthy controls. It turned out that the two facets of alexithymia prominent in DDD, *difficulty identifying* (DIF) and *difficulty describing* (DDF) feelings, were subsumed by *distinct* altered neural responses (plus, brain areas responsible for processing happy vs. sad emotions are not the same). When DDD participants processed *happy* faces, DIF was linked to right anterior insula activity and DDF to right anterior cingulate activity. For *sad* faces, DIF was linked to left anterior insula activity and DDF to right posterior cingulate activity. The *insula* is central to the *interoception* and identification of our emotions (the way it feels inside when we are happy, or sad). The *cingulate* cortex is central to *monitoring* and *reflecting* on any emotion sensed inside, so that we can describe and express it. Simply put, the study identified neural substrates associated with both components of alexithymia in DDD, distinct for sensing and expressing emotion.

Lastly, neuroimaging studies involving PTSD rather than DDD have compared "classic" PTSD to the "dissociative subtype" of PTSD.[23] As we've already discussed, the dissociative subtype is distinguished from PTSD as usual by the presence of persistent dpdr (see the latest edition of the *Diagnostic and Statistical Manual of Mental Disorders* [DSM-5-TR] and Chapter 5). The former group, when presented with traumatic reminders, experienced intense arousal, increased heart rate, and flashbacks, whereas the latter group shut down and did not experience an increase in arousal and heart rate.

The two groups' brain activation patterns, examined with fMRI while the participants were exposed to personalized traumatic scripts, appeared very different. The dissociative PTSD group had increased brain activation in the medial prefrontal cortex and the anterior cingulate cortex (both involved in cognitive processing and inhibition of emotional responses), as well as increased brain activity in sensory association areas of the temporal, parietal, and occipital lobes. These patterns are consistent with both the *sensory association cortex* and *cortico-limbic disconnection* models that we've explored in the first two sections in relation to DDD.

The Autonomic System

Neuroscience research has established that there is bidirectional communication between limbic regions and the autonomic system; the two systems work together to regulate the experiencing and expression of emotions. The autonomic system is the part of the nervous system that regulates basic organ processes necessary for the maintenance of normal bodily functions, such as heart rate and blood pressure, and is of particular interest in dissociation. In some psychiatric disorders associated with high levels of anxiety and arousal, such as panic disorder and PTSD, the autonomic system is hyperreactive. In contrast, in dissociative conditions and states the autonomic system tends to be hyporeactive. For example, women who experience dissociation after being raped have decreased autonomic (heart rate and skin conductance) responses.[24] Using a method known as skin conductance, one can study the peripheral autonomic system and its response to arousing stimuli. In effect, the skin momentarily becomes a better conductor of electricity when a person is aroused by internal or external stimuli.

Hypoemotionality is one of the core features of DDD, and there is compelling evidence for autonomic system hyporeactivity in the disorder. One study measuring skin conductance response (SCR) reported that DDD participants had decreased SCR, compared to people with anxiety disorders and healthy individuals, in response to emotionally unpleasant pictures; no differences were found in response to pleasant pictures. In other words, the DDD group was less aroused by and responsive to negative emotional stimuli, yet did not show diminished SCR to nonspecific arousing stimuli such as the sound of a clap—the observed phenomenon was a *selective inhibition of emotionality*.[25] A subsequent SCR study used the same two comparison groups and examined DDD autonomic responses to emotional facial expressions. The three groups did not differ in their SCR responses to happy faces, but when it came to disgusted faces, the DDD group had a similar autonomic reaction to healthy controls, while anxious patients had a heightened response.[26] These two SCR studies are important for a reason additional to linking DDD hypoemotionality to autonomic hyporeactivity: DDD and anxiety disorder responses differed in both studies, suggesting that dpdr cannot be adequately conceptualized as an anxiety variant.

Dr. Matthias Michal, a DDD researcher based in Germany, and colleagues examined the impact of mindful breathing on the autonomic responses to emotional sounds, positive and negative ones.[27] DDD patients were compared to a mixed patient group with similar depression and anxiety. The study found that in the baseline listening condition (no mindful breathing), DDD patients responded more strongly (SCR) to all emotional sounds, especially the negative ones. However, in the mindful condition, DDD patients were better able to modulate their response to emotional sounds, in a similar way to controls, and at the same time experienced a reduction in dpdr and felt more grounded. This finding may have treatment implications (see Chapter 11), as patients cannot engage as effectively in the psychotherapy process when they are in more extreme states of emotional arousal, be it overarousal or underarousal.

The autonomic system has two major components, the *sympathetic* and the *parasympathetic* nervous systems (SNS and PNS respectively). Whereas the SNS mediates responses to stress, the widely known fight-or-flight response, the PNS has a dampening effect and regulates functioning during quiescence and rest. The SNS uses norepinephrine, an adrenaline-like substance, as its chemical messenger. Norepinephrine facilitates alertness, orientation toward new stimuli, selective attention, and enhanced memory encoding under stressful conditions, in the service of survival and adaptation. However, although bursts in norepinephrine activity under acute stress are adaptive, more chronic noradrenergic activation "for no good reason," such as that encountered in certain psychiatric conditions related to traumatic stress, is maladaptive. For example, several studies have shown a heightened noradrenergic tone in people with PTSD, which goes hand in hand with the hyperarousal and intrusive symptoms.

Dissociative states are, in this sense, the "opposite" of classic PTSD. Instead of hyperarousal there is "shutdown," so one would predict noradrenergic dysregulation of an opposite sort. In fact, three studies have found a relationship between dissociation and lower norepinephrine levels. Dr. Simeon's group found that in people with DDD, the norepinephrine level in a urine sample collected over 24 hours was inversely related to dissociation severity; in other words, the stronger the dissociation, the lower the norepinephrine.[28] The researchers found this same inverse relationship between dissociation severity and 24-hour urine norepinephrine levels in a group of patients with borderline personality disorder who had varying degrees of dissociation.[29] A similar finding was reported in the immediate aftermath of car accidents: urine norepinephrine levels were inversely related to the victims' peritraumatic dissociation severity.[30]

Finally, what is the role of the *parasympathetic* system in DDD? As we already said, this system is activated in states of calm, and brings about the shutting down of the *sympathetic* nervous system response once an acute stressor ends. Practices such as meditation, deep breathing, yoga, relaxation, pleasant visualizations, and even play activate the system—as we all know from personal experience. Though inhibition of the SNS is better established in DDD, as we just discussed, the PNS had received little attention until a 2015 publication by Dr. Owens and colleagues in the British group.[31] DDD and healthy participants were compared in their heart rate variability response to a standard cardiovascular tilt maneuver while viewing a constant stream of unpleasant pictures (the cardiovascular system is tightly regulated by both the SNS and the PNS, and heart rate variability is an indicator of PNS activity). The study found that the DDD group was not able to mobilize the PNS as effectively as the comparison group, and so dampen their reactivity to the negative images, while being cardiovascularly stressed.

In summary, DDD patients appear to have a mix of both sympathetic and parasympathetic dysregulation, which may differ for nonspecific physiological arousal versus specific emotional arousal and, additionally, vary within the context of a restful or stressed state. These patterns are rather reminiscent of the emotional cognition findings described in the previous chapter: at baseline DDD participants recalled fewer negative words than healthy controls, yet after stress they remembered them more—when aroused, it was harder to shut down the "negative."

The Hypothalamic-Pituitary-Adrenal Axis

The hypothalamic-pituitary-adrenal (HPA) axis is a neurohormonal system key to regulating our response to stress. The circuit works as follows (Figure 8.3).

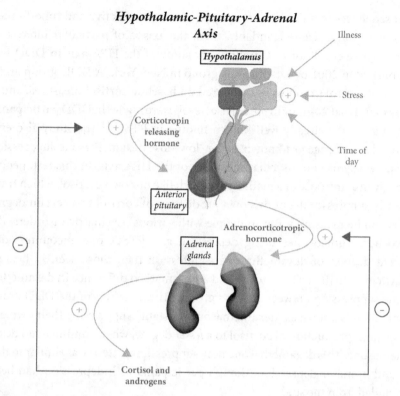

Figure 8.3 Diagram of the hypothalamic-pituitary-adrenal axis.
(Source: joshya/Shutterstock.)

A brainstem structure known as the hypothalamus is activated by stress and secretes corticotrophin-releasing hormone (CRF); CRF, in turn, activates the brain's pituitary gland to secrete adrenocorticotropic hormone (ACTH), which in turn stimulates our adrenal glands to secrete the stress hormone cortisol. Cortisol has widespread actions throughout the body and the brain via the glucocorticoid receptors, mounting an immediate stress response that effectively mobilizes necessary body and brain responses while shutting down energy-wasting responses that are a "luxury" in the face of acute stress (e.g., digestion). In the end, via a closed loop, cortisol is also responsible for shutting down the acute stress response, by its negative feedback inhibition of the pituitary and the hypothalamus. The HPA axis normally functions like a fine-tuned, self-contained, and self-regulating stress-response system.

However, in psychiatric conditions linked to early life adversity or later severe stress and trauma, the HPA axis can go haywire, with detrimental consequences to a person's capacity to mount an effective and time-limited stress response. Understandably, then, the axis is of particular interest in dissociative conditions. A preliminary study of the HPA axis in DDD was published in 2001 by Dr. Simeon's group in New York. A DDD group and a healthy control group were compared on baseline cortisol measures, and it was found that 24-hour urine cortisol levels were higher in DDD participants, *opposite* to the already well-known finding in PTSD.[32] The study also employed a challenge test known as the "low-dose dexamethasone suppression test," widely used in psychiatric studies of the HPA axis. In this test, people are given a tiny dose of a medication much like our own cortisol, which transiently suppresses the body's own production of cortisol to a certain degree that can be measured. But in people with various psychiatric disorders, the two best-studied ones being depression and PTSD, one encounters different degrees of dexamethasone suppression than those seen in healthy participants. The DDD study found a very marked difference in dexamethasone suppression between the two groups. The members of the DDD group were what is known as "dexamethasone resistant," suppressing their own endogenous production of cortisol to a *lesser* degree, when administered dexamethasone. This dexamethasone non-suppression pattern was similar to that found in major depression, though participants with depression had been excluded from the study.

The investigators moved on to a larger and more definitive study to find out HPA axis function in DDD; their findings were published six years later in the journal *Biological Psychiatry*.[33] (Note that the HPA axis had already been extensively studied in PTSD and characterized as "hypersensitive;" the research team hypothesized that a converse pattern of sorts might occur in a dissociative disorder not associated with PTSD.) This new study involved 46 DDD patients, 35 with PTSD, and 58 healthy controls. The first phase consisted of a 24-hour urine collection and hourly blood sampling to measure baseline levels of cortisol—cortisol is a diurnal hormone highly sensitive to time of day. In the second phase, the low-dose dexamethasone suppression test described earlier was administered. In the third phase, participants underwent the Trier Social Stress Test (TSST) and their cortisol response was measured. The TSST is a standardized experimental method used to study the impact of psychosocial stress, and has been used in various psychiatric studies. Participants are asked to stand in front of a solemn and expressionless small group of "judges" and perform certain tasks (math and a mock interview) as best they can, believing that their performance is being graded.

The results were illuminating, replicating and expanding the findings of the earlier study. First, the DDD group had elevated urinary cortisol levels compared to healthy controls, in fact more pronounced in the absence of lifetime major depression, whereas the PTSD and healthy control groups did not differ from each other. Second, the DDD group demonstrated significantly greater resistance to, and faster escape from, dexamethasone suppression compared to the healthy control group, whereas the PTSD and healthy control groups did not differ. Third, although the three groups did not differ in cortisol reactivity to the TSST (naturally, the stressful test increased cortisol secretion in all), both psychiatric groups demonstrated a significant inverse relationship between dissociation severity and cortisol reactivity, after controlling for all other symptoms. In other words, the more dissociated a patient, the lesser the cortisol surge in response to stress—an insufficient stress response was mounted. All in all, this study demonstrated a distinctive pattern of HPA axis dysregulation in DDD, both supporting the role of traumatic stress in the genesis of the disorder, and accounting for the perpetuation of vulnerability to stress.

Is There a Link to Serotonin?

Several experts in the field, including Sir Martin Roth, Dr. Eric Hollander, and Dr. Evan Torch (see Chapter 2), had noted how depersonalization can sometimes look like a variant of obsessive-compulsive disorder (OCD). As we've already discussed earlier in the book, some DDD patients present with an obsessive-compulsive type of elaboration of their dpdr experiences. They may incessantly ruminate and obsess about what it is like to have no self, about life being real or a dream, the nature of existence, and all the possible implications of their symptoms. Checking rituals often accompany these ruminations.

This phenomenon poses the question of whether the "obsessive-compulsive" presentation is inherent to the underlying brain dysfunction of DDD, part and parcel of feeling unreal, or an elaboration that occurs only in DDD people who are prone to obsessionality. There is certainly a substantial subgroup that engages in this nonproductive and torturous "thinking in circles," but it's important to remember that there are many others with DDD who do not. Sometimes, as we've seen, this type of thinking can occur in the earlier stages of the condition and can even be a "defensive" attempt to understand and make sense of the experience of unreality, later flattening out into emotional deadness and a reluctantly accepted state of "no self."

An inherent obsessive-compulsive component to DDD would suggest that serotonergic dysfunction might play a role in the genesis of the disorder, since the neurotransmitter serotonin is well known to play a role in OCD and related disorders. However, data supporting this hypothesis are rather limited. One indirect source of evidence is the fact that depersonalized states can be transiently induced in healthy people by hallucinogens, such as LSD, psilocybin, and DMT, in both naturalistic and experimental settings (see next chapter). Regarding DDD, about 6% of a cohort of 117 DDD patients reported precipitation of chronic dpdr by acute hallucinogen use.[34] Hallucinogens, in fact, act as agonists (enhance neurotransmission) of the serotonin 5HT2 A and C receptors, possibly suggesting a mediating role for serotonin.

One study, by Drs. Simeon and Hollander, examined a mixed group of non-DDD participants (social anxiety disorder, OCD, borderline personality disorder, and healthy controls), in whom transient dpdr and other symptoms were induced with a one-time dose of either meta-chlorophenylpiperazine (mCPP), an experimental serotonin agonist, or placebo.[35] mCPP administration elicited a much higher rate of dpdr in this diverse group than placebo did, although it also induced more anxiety, panic, and dysphoria as well—in other words, the effect might have been nonspecific. Similarly, Dr. Southwick and colleagues reported that when mCPP was administered to a PTSD group, the serotonergic activation induced flashbacks and dissociative symptoms in a subgroup of participants[36] (unfortunately, PTSD dissociative subtype did not officially exist back then as a designated subgroup in the *DSM*). So, while these are not particularly clean models for *pure* depersonalization, they do suggest that serotonin may play a modulating role in DDD.

Consistent with the limited evidence for a serotonin hypothesis in DDD, selective serotonin reuptake inhibitor medications (SSRIs—fluoxetine, sertraline, and the like) are not highly effective in treating the disorder, especially in the absence of co-occurring anxiety, depression, or OCD (see Chapter 10). This fact negates a central role for a serotonergic hypothesis of DDD. The degree to which SSRIs, or other classes of antidepressants such as tricyclics and monoamine oxidase inhibitors (MAOIs), "leach" into other neurochemical pathways modulated by serotonin, or indirectly help dpdr through a decrease in associated anxiety or depression, may be reasons why these drugs are of some benefit in a number of DDD sufferers.

The Endogenous Opioid System

There are three endogenous opioid systems (EOSs) in the brain— the mu, kappa, and delta systems. Both the mu and the kappa systems have been, to some degree, implicated in dpdr. Stress-induced analgesia (diminished pain sensitivity) is known to be mediated by the mu EOS. For example, in veterans suffering from combat-related PTSD, the analgesic response to combat scenes can be blocked by pretreatment with the opioid antagonist naloxone.[37] With respect to the kappa opioid system, the pure kappa opioid agonist enadoline was shown to induce a "clean" depersonalization-like syndrome in healthy subjects, compared to placebo, with perceptual disturbances and a sense of detachment as the main manifestations.[38]

Along these lines, "nonselective" opiate antagonists, ones that block all three types of EOS receptors when used in high enough dosages, have been reported to reduce dissociation in a few studies. This has been shown, for example, with high-dose naltrexone treatment in borderline personality disorder, as well as intravenous naloxone or oral naltrexone treatment in chronic dpdr (we will be talking more about these treatments in Chapter 10). Selective opioid antagonists that block only the kappa receptors have been of some interest in the treatment of psychiatric disorders for years now but are still in the pharmaceutical development "pipeline," and have not yet reached the market.

Gray Matter

The brain consists of gray and white matter—gray matter is made up of neuronal cell bodies, whereas white matter is made out of nerve fibers. Simply put, the gray matter is where brain processing occurs, while white matter transmits information between areas of gray matter. Volumetric imaging studies examine only the structure of the brain, essentially determining whether the gray matter is intact or altered in volume from the normative. Though brain structure does not directly translate into brain function (for example, a region of gray matter might be smaller, but its functions may be compensated for by other brain areas), volumetric measurements can be meaningful by pointing us in the direction of possible functional abnormalities.

Investigations of whole-brain gray matter aberrations in the dissociative disorders are limited in the medical literature. A few older studies focused exclusively on amygdalar, hippocampal, and parahippocampal gray matter volumes mainly in dissociative identity disorder and did not include patients with DDD. However, in 2015, a structural MRI whole-brain study was published, comparing 25 patients with DDD to 23 healthy controls.[39] The DDD group turned out to have significant gray matter volume *decreases* in the right caudate, the right thalamus, and the right middle and superior occipital gyri. Conversely, significant volume *increases* in the DDD group involved the left medial superior frontal gyrus, the right superior temporal gyrus, and the right parietal postcentral gyrus (notably, the amygdala and hippocampus did not differ in size between the two groups).

What could these findings mean or implicate in terms of DDD brain function? In a structural study, findings are more compelling when they can be shown to be related to some manifest aspect of the condition being studied, for example the severity of symptoms. And, in fact, within the DDD group the investigators reported a significant relationship between gray matter volume alterations and dpdr severity, suggesting that the structural changes were relevant to the expression of the disorder. Furthermore, two of the areas with altered volume were the same brain areas that were found to have altered brain activity in the DDD PET imaging study described earlier: the superior occipital gyrus (BA 19) and the superior temporal gyrus (BA 22), both sensory association areas in the posterior brain.

The thalamus is the brain's gateway for sensory input, relaying sensory information to corresponding cortical areas—as we discussed earlier with regard to the thalamo-cortical dysconnectivity model. And synchronized brain wave activity between the thalamus and the cortex is believed to mediate the *conscious* awareness of sensory and emotional experiences. The caudate receives input from cortical emotion processing areas, and in turn projects back to the thalamus. The study, then, might suggest that the normal communication loops between the thalamus, specific cortical areas, and the caudate are disrupted in DDD, and subsume the dpdr experiences. In particular, the areas identified by the study are thought to be associated with phenomena such as subjective body ownership (thalamus and caudate); motion and depth perception (occipital areas); executive control of attention and emotion (frontal area); and proprioception (parietal area).

Brain Rhythms

In 2020, an exciting and potentially important paper was published in the journal *Nature*, conducted by a Stanford research group headed by renowned neuroscientist Karl Deisseroth and graduate students Sam Vesuna, PhD, and Isaac Kauvar, PhD.[40] This research group believes it may have identified a key and novel neural circuit involved in dissociation, as well as its molecular underpinnings. Though the study was conducted in mice, not humans, the mice findings were echoed in the case of one patient with chronic epilepsy, also included in the report. As in a best-case scenario for any neuroscience "discovery," the group suggested that the findings might "translate" into novel treatment approaches for dissociation, because they implicate a particular protein within a particular group of brain cells.

Let's start with the bulk of the study, the mice experiments. Ketamine is a "dissociative anesthetic" that readers are familiar with by now: recall Dr. Krystal's corticocortical and thalamo-cortical dysconnectivity, ketamine-centered, model from over two decades ago, earlier in this chapter. In the experiments by Deisseroth's group, mice were administered a ketamine dose that appeared to induce dissociation. Since mice cannot directly communicate their feelings or states-of-mind, inferences were made from their behavior. The mice acted in ways that suggested they were dissociated: there seemed to be a "disconnect" between what they were sensing and perceiving, and their emotional and behavioral responses to these inputs. In one example, the mice behaved differently than they usually do when placed on an unpleasantly warm surface: normally they don't like it, and they habitually flick and lick their paws to cool down. However, under the influence of ketamine, this behavioral response was eliminated: it was as if the mice couldn't care less about the uncomfortable sensations, and since they were not emotionally affected they did not bother to engage in cooling-down. Similar dissociative states were induced in the mice using phencyclidine (better known as "angel dust"), a hallucinogenic anesthetic.

Precisely where this altered experience sits in the brain needed to be located. Using a technique known as optogenetics, the researchers found that a very particular section (layer 5) of a very particular cortical region (the retrosplenial cortex) was firing at a very particular rhythm (1 to 3 Hz), in the dissociative state induced by the two drugs. Furthermore, though this rhythm was coupled with the rhythm of the part of the thalamus relaying signals to the retrosplenial cortex, it was uncoupled from the portion of the thalamus that projects to the frontal lobes. Lastly, the specific "dissociative" rhythm was induced by ketamine's action on a particular potassium channel (HCN1) in the affected neurons.

The retrosplenial cortex (BA 29 and 30) and its connections to other parts of the brain are thought to be conserved across mammals (i.e., the mice findings may extend to humans). It sits deep in the posterior part of the brain and has rich connections to the hippocampus, the limbic (emotional) part of the thalamus, and the parietal cortex. Still, do these dissociation findings truly translate to humans? It is important that a study like this, putting forth a novel physiological and molecular model for dissociation, say something about humans; and indeed the article included an illustrative case of a patient with chronic epilepsy. This patient experienced dissociation immediately before each seizure; the dissociative "aura" felt "like being outside the pilot's chair, looking at, but not controlling, the gauges"—depersonalization, for sure, with disembodiment and diminished agency.

The research group recorded electrical activity from various brain regions in this patient, who had electrodes implanted in order to better localize seizure activity and offer effective treatment. It turned out this individual's dissociation (when it occurred spontaneously and was electrically recorded) was associated with the same 3-Hz rhythm in the deep posteromedial cortex—a human brain region analogous to the mouse retrosplenial cortex. And, the same exact pattern was replicated when the team electrically stimulated this region: the person experienced the exact same dissociation, though without a seizure.

Although it is premature to draw definitive conclusions from a single human, this study may prove to be a landmark one, if replicated, extended, and translated to human research. Could it be that a particular low-frequency rhythm, hidden deep in the retrosplenial/posteromedial cortex, is an evolutionarily conserved mechanism that underlies dissociation across species? Time will, hopefully, teach us more about the neuroscience of altered consciousness.

Neuroscience of Selfhood

We have reviewed much of the known neuroscience relating to key components of DDD. But what about the core sense of selfhood, which in DDD can be so greatly disrupted that some patients describe that they have *no self?* Unreality and hypoemotionality are certainly parts of this "selfless-ness," but they may not be the whole story.

An experimental method known as the self-face paradigm has been used in neuroscience studies to examine the neural foundations of the self. In 2014, Drs. Ketay and Simeon undertook such a study in DDD to better un-derstand the neurobiology of the "unfamiliar self."[41] The study compared a DDD group with a healthy control group, as all participants underwent fMRI while viewing photographs of their own faces and a stranger's face that was matched to their own face in basic characteristics. The study found that compared to controls, DDD patients exhibited greater activation when pro-cessing images of the self, versus the stranger, in three brain regions: the right anterior cingulate, the bilateral medial prefrontal cortex, and the left middle frontal gyrus. Furthermore, depersonalization severity was correlated with activity in the latter two brain regions. What could these findings mean?

It turns out that the *medial prefrontal cortex* has been consistently implicated in neuroimaging studies of self-versus-other judgments conducted in healthy volunteers. The greater activation of this area in DDD could reflect the difficulty in experiencing one's face with a sense of owner-ship and familiarity. The investigators also offered an intriguing potential ex-planation for the activation of the *anterior cingulate*. This part of the brain is central to conflict resolution. It might, therefore, have been activated because of the conflict generated in DDD participants, who on one hand "know" their own face, but on the other hand don't quite "know" it: is it my face or isn't it? A similar activation pattern has been reported in another dissociative condition, conversion disorder.

Clearly, the neurobiological underpinnings of the self, and of conscious-ness, are among the most challenging frontiers in modern neuroscience, and we can expect to see more such studies in DDD, the quintessential psychi-atric disorder characterized by subjectively altered consciousness and loss of selfhood.

9

The Blow of the Void and Spirituality

If the doors of perception were cleansed, everything would appear to man as it is, infinite.

—William Blake

Though its exploration as a disorder is more recent, feelings of depersonalization and derealization have been expressed in many ways for centuries. Struggling with this mental change can lead down many paths, sometimes implying a spiritual awakening unknown to those with depersonalization/derealization disorder (DDD), often leading to anxiety and fruitless rumination and, on occasion, works of art. Like the literary figure of Satan, its enigmatic face has surfaced under many names, and many guises—one only need know where to look.

Alienation, isolation, and altered perceptions have been longstanding themes for the visual arts, particularly modern art. Edvard Munch's famous painting "The Scream" depicts the essence of a private hell severed from the world. Vincent Van Gogh's frenetically intense stars invite the depths of the galaxy into our world. In the twentieth century, Surrealists challenged the concrete representations of our reality—Salvador Dali's warped clocks don't track time, and René Magritte's hyperreal pipe questions its existence as such ("Ceci n'est pas une pipe"). Whether stemming from the altered consciousness of mental afflictions or the saner calculated play with all that we take for granted, the boundaries of the real and the unreal are momentarily suspended in those who are touched by the iconic works of master painters.

Detachment, estrangement, alienation, as well as a heightened and troubling awareness of the infinite and the eternal, also appear in written works, from the Bible, to Shakespeare, to Dostoevsky, to modern pop lyrics. Yet all the former may or may not involve depersonalization per se, which has also specifically had its place in the arts and in philosophy. As early as the 1600s

Feeling Unreal. Second Edition. Daphne Simeon and Jeffrey Abugel, Oxford University Press. © Oxford University Press 2023. DOI: 10.1093/oso/9780197622445.003.0009

philosopher Blaise Pascal articulated the kind of existential realization that often accompanies depersonalization:

> When I consider the short duration of my life, swallowed up in the eternity before and after, the little space which I fill, and even can see—engulfed in an infinite immensity of spaces of which I am ignorant and which know me not, I am frightened, and am astonished at being here rather than there, for there is no reason why here rather than there, why now rather than then. The eternal silence of these infinite spaces frightens me.[1]

Of course, in a purely philosophical sense, such observations may be relatively fleeting, and familiar to any reflective or "deep" thinker. They simply resonate with depersonalized people to a greater degree. The essential library more directly related to depersonalization includes a surprisingly diverse group of books and stories that are all loosely interwoven by common themes.

The First Depersonalization Diary

The book from which Ludovic Dugas drew the name for his subject of investigation serves as a fitting starting point. This was Henri Frédéric Amiel's private diary, *Journal Intime*.[2] Amiel's journal is one of literature's great curiosities. Published posthumously in 1882, it is the private diary of an obscure Swiss university professor who lived from 1821 to 1881. Day by day, over a period of more than 30 years, Amiel documented his most intimate thoughts and observations on many subjects, including European culture, politics, religion, women, and, in particular, his own identity. In all, Amiel penned more than 17,000 journal entries.

Before his death, Amiel requested that his friends, who included several writers and literary critics, find some use for his voluminous journal. The result was a condensed two-volume work that has earned a unique place in the annals of psychology and philosophy. Amiel's *Journal* does not reveal a solitary thinker's slow descent into madness as some had expected. It is, instead, the meticulous record of a man whose life never really got off the ground because he was never really grounded in this life. He was, using his terminology, from the age of 16, depersonalized.

Amiel was born to French parents in Geneva, Switzerland, where he lived and worked his entire life. When he was 12 years old, both of his parents died while in their 30s. Living with relatives, he was understandably forlorn and melancholic and showed a deep interest in religious ideas, particularly Calvinism, which was prevalent in Geneva at the time. As he matured, he traveled widely and was exposed to the most prominent of the nineteenth century's thinkers, including Rousseau and Hegel. He completed his formal education in Heidelberg and Berlin, then returned home. Amid the continent's social upheavals, Geneva provided a peaceful haven for someone like Amiel, who showed potential for contributing to the rapidly evolving political, philosophical, and scientific thinking of the day.

He began a promising career by winning a public competition to become professor of French literature at the prestigious Academy of Geneva. Just four years later, at age 28, he was elevated to professor of moral philosophy, on the fast track to traditional academic success. For Amiel, however, the prestigious job in academia was not a fortuitous beginning but a dead end. In time, as the years passed, his friends and acquaintances began to wonder why. He was uncommonly intelligent, articulate, even sociable, yet year after year, nothing emerged from this wellspring of possibilities but dry college lectures and, periodically, literary criticism that reaffirmed his talent, followed by poetry that did not.

His closest confidant, critic M. Edmund Scherer, recalled years later: "He awakened in us but one regret; we could not understand how it was a man so richly gifted produced nothing, or only trivialities" (p. xxii).[2] The answer all along, unknown to his friends, was recorded in his private journal, which spawned keen interest, particularly from an unexpected quarter—the leading psychologists of the day. The journal was something yet unseen, a lifelong case history of a certain type of personality, which could be excerpted out of context to prove a point for any number of emerging psychological theories. To Dugas he was detached and depersonalized, to Pierre Janet he likely manifested "psychasthenia" and its characteristic *sentiment d'incompletude* (sense of incompleteness), and still others saw his life as incorporating an unlikely combination of Christian and Buddhist belief systems. But above all, his writing reflects a personal life that is symptomatic of the indecision and dysfunction so often associated with chronic depersonalization.

Amiel's depersonalization did not often manifest itself in numbness or lack of feeling; he felt things deeply. But a predominant theme permeates his journal: the world and everything in it, including his personal identity, felt unreal, unfounded, and without substance. True reality, he concluded, beyond the veil of the day-to-day world, consisted of the eternal, the infinite, God. The more the self dissolved, the closer one came to the truth and to God, he rationalized. Theologically, these are not original thoughts and are shared by Buddhists, Hindus, and certain New Age theosophists of today. But Amiel's conclusions are not the result of meditation or religious training. He feels the absence of an individual Self, and, at times, this translates into an elusive but heartfelt connection with the Infinite. While he eloquently voices the importance of this distinctly non-European point of view, one is not always sure whether he is trying to convince the reader or himself.

"Be everything while being nothing," he writes early in the journal, "effacing thyself, letting God enter into thee as the air enters an empty vessel, reducing the ego to the mere vessel which contains the divine essence." Yet most of his language is less preachy—less a justification of the empty feeling he is unable to shake. Reflecting on an afternoon meeting with some fellow intellectuals, Amiel makes a keen observation that is more typical of his prose: "Nothing is more hidden from us than the illusion which lives with us day by day, and our greatest illusion is to believe that we are what we think ourselves to be."

While many of Amiel's written observations are highly quotable and are used by writers and scholars to this day, his journal consistently and eloquently expresses the experience of chronic, lifelong depersonalization above all else. In this regard, Amiel's story is best captured by excerpts from his journal:

> I can find no words for what I feel. My consciousness is withdrawn into itself; I hear my heart beating, and my life passing. It seems to me that I have become a statue on the banks of the river of time, that I am the spectator of some mystery, and shall issue from it old, or no longer capable of age. . . . I am a spectator, so to speak, of the molecular whirlwind which men call individual life; I am conscious of an incessant metamorphosis; an irresistible movement of existence, which is going on within me—and this phenomenology of myself serves as a window opened upon the mystery of the world . . . What is it which has always come between real life and me? What glass screen has, as it were, interposed itself between me and the enjoyment, the possession, the contact of things, leaving me only the role of the looker-on? False shame, no doubt. I have been ashamed to desire. Fatal results of timidity, aggravated by intellectual delusion! Fear, too, has had

a large share in it—*la peur de ce que j'aime est ma fatalité* [the fear of what I love is my fate].

This sentiment in many ways reflects the experience of some chronically depersonalized people, whose robotic actions stem from inhibitions like Amiel's fear and shame. They desire to act and appear normal lest bursts of desire, creativity, eccentricity, or iconoclastic behavior seem symptomatic of insanity or reveal to others the dreaded secret of a mental problem. As a result, many depersonalized people live in a more phobic and constricted way than they might otherwise have. For Amiel, robot-like behavior is a matter of going through the motions of his job and private literary exercises that never blossom into a literary statement beyond the confines of his journal.

In the 1880s, Amiel began to express frustration at the lack of achievement that resulted from his obsessive self-examination:

> I am afraid of greatness. All my published literary essays, therefore, are little else than studies, games, exercises, for the purpose of testing myself. I play scales, as it were: I run up and down my instrument, I train my hand, and make sure of its capacity and skill. But the work itself remains unachieved. My effort expires, and satisfied with the power to act, I never arrive at the will to act, I am always preparing and never accomplishing and my energy is swallowed up in a kind of barren curiosity . . . I understand myself, but I do not approve myself.

Unfortunately for this gentle, sensitive man, instead of being instilled by his intelligence and insight with a sense of confidence and faith, his chronic introspection brought only loneliness, regret, and self-contradiction. He fills the journal with some entries that praise the value of ego-death, while other entries decry his lack of ambition and motivation and the mediocrity of his accomplishments in the academic and literary world. This dichotomy between earthly ambition and selfless, eternal unification with God locked him in a kind of "analysis paralysis" his entire life. He became a fussy perfectionist, and because he couldn't write the perfect novel, he didn't write one at all. Because he couldn't find the perfect wife, he never married. And through it all, he obsessed about existence itself, convinced of how little his life in the world mattered because he never really felt himself to be part of it.

Mrs. Humphrey (Mary Augusta) Ward, a noted literary and humanitarian woman of the time, and the translator of Amiel's work, says in her 1885
introduction:

> There were certain characteristics in Amiel which made it [success]
> impossible—which neutralized his powers, his knowledge, his intelligence,
> and condemned him, so far as his public performance was concerned, to bar
> renness and failure. . . . All of the pleasant paths which traverse the kingdom
> of Knowledge, in which so many of us find shelter and life-long means of
> happiness, led Amiel straight into the wilderness of abstract speculation.

So much was true. But his journal also revealed an exceptional degree of
self-awareness, honesty, and truth. In May 1880, Amiel wrote:

> I have lived the impersonal life—in the world, yet not in it, thinking much,
> desiring nothing. It is a state of mind which corresponds with what in
> women is called a broken heart; and it is in fact like it, since the character
> istic common to both is despair. When one knows that one will never pos
> sess what one could have loved, and that one can be content with nothing
> less, one has, so to speak, left the world, one has cut the golden hair, parted
> with all that makes human life—that is to say, illusion—the incessant effort
> towards an apparently attainable end.

Amiel is virtually incapable of the self-deceptions that people often utilize
for survival or in striving toward worldly goals with a sense of agency. It has
been impossible for him to playact in a day-to-day world that feels unreal and
pointless. Near the end of some 30 years of philosophical comments, in his
50s, Amiel provides the reader with some important insight into the origins
of his enduring state of mind:

> Since the age of 16 onwards I have been able to look at things with the eyes
> of a blind man recently operated upon. That is to say, I have been able to
> suppress in myself the results of the long education of sight, and to abolish
> distances; and now I find myself regarding existence as though from be
> yond the tomb, from another world; all is strange to me; I am, as it were,
> outside my own body and individuality; I am *depersonalized*, detached, cut
> adrift. Is this madness? No. Madness means the impossibility of recovering
> one's normal balance after the mind has thus played truant among alien

forms of being, and followed Dante to invisible worlds. Madness means in-capacity for self-judgement and self-control. Whereas it seems to me that my mental transformations are but philosophical experiences.

In the above paragraph, Amiel unintentionally gives birth to the term that is the subject of this book, while at the same time demonstrating the "in-tact reality testing" that also marks the condition. Ludovic Dugas and others, picking up on the term that fit so well with their Amiel-like patients, gave a condition yet unnamed its moniker. As psychiatrist J. C. Nemiah said:

What is of particular interest in the journal entry quoted [above] is Amiel's awareness that his capacity for insight into his condition was maintained throughout all the alterations of his perceptions of himself and the world. He also recognized that no matter how bizarre his experiences were, the preservation of insight kept them clearly out of the realm of madness. . . . Amiel's perceptive introspection revealed to him a clinical truth about de-personalization that remains a central element of the modern concept of the disorder: patients have a keen and unfailing awareness of the disturbances in their sense of reality. . . . There appears in depersonalization to be a heightening of the psychic energy invested in the self-observing ego, the mental function on which rests the capacity for insight.[3]

Dr. Elena Bezzubova has aptly summed the paradox of Amiel's life: "Amiel's fear to begin, to accomplish, really a fear of being himself is a kernel of the self while at the same time the root of self-decay. . . . Reality's static, half-true na-ture is deathlike. But searching for reality as a permanent process can also kill, dissolving the self into particles of estrangement" (personal communication). Regardless of Amiel's ultimate fulfillment or disillusionment with his life, he and others who followed did capture, as close as language permits in poignant and ethereal prose, the essence of depersonalized existence—offering great comfort to others who strive to put their own confounding experiences into words.

Behind the Cotton Wool

For some, writing is the only real way to express, or attempt to make sense of, anomalous mental experiences. Virginia Woolf, who suffered from lifelong mental illness, revealed instances of what she called "wool" as the concealing fabric of day-to-day-life and reminiscent of Amiel's "glass screen"—a division between reality and unreality, the seen and unseen.

Woolf described "moments of being"—moments in which an individual experiences a sense of reality—in contrast to the states of "non-being" that dominate most of an individual's conscious life, in which they are separated from reality by a protective covering. It is, for her, at least a partial cleansing of the doors of perception. She describes three instances wherein sudden realizations, "blows," consume her consciousness to reveal true being.[4]

I was fighting with Thoby [Woolf's older brother] on the lawn. We were pommeling each other with our fists. Just as I raised my fist to hit him, I felt: why hurt another person? I dropped my hand instantly, and stood there, and let him beat me. I remember the feeling. It was a feeling of hopeless sadness. It was as if I became aware of something terrible; and of my own powerlessness. I slunk off alone, feeling horribly depressed. The second instance was also in the garden at St Ives. I was looking at the flower bed by the front door; "That is the whole," I said. I was looking at a plant with a spread of leaves; and it seemed suddenly plain that the flower itself was a part of the earth; that a ring enclosed what was the flower; and that was the real flower; part earth; part flower. The third case was also at St Ives. Some people called Valpy had been staying at St Ives, and had left. We were waiting at dinner one night, when somehow I overheard my father or my mother say that Mr Valpy had killed himself. The next thing I remember is being in the garden at night and walking on the path by the apple tree. It seemed to me that the apple tree was connected with the horror of Mr Valpy's suicide. I could not pass it. I stood there looking at the grey-green creases of the bark—it was a moonlit night—in a trance of horror. I seemed to be dragged down, hopelessly, into some pit of absolute despair from which I could not escape. My body seemed paralysed.

These were three instances of exceptional moments . . . Two of these moments ended in a state of despair. The other ended, on the contrary, in a state of satisfaction. When I said about the flower "That is the whole," I felt that I had made a discovery . . . It strikes me now that this was a profound difference. It was the difference in the first place between despair and satisfaction. This difference I think arose from the fact that I was quite unable to deal with the pain of discovering that people hurt each other, that a man I had seen had killed himself. The sense of horror held me powerless. But in the case of the flower I found a reason; and was thus able to deal with the sensation. I was not powerless. I was conscious—if only at a distance—that I should in time explain it.

I hazard the explanation that a shock is at once in my case followed by the desire to explain it. I feel that I have had a blow; but it is not, as I thought as a child, simply a blow from an enemy hidden behind the cotton wool of daily life; it is or will become a revelation of some order; it is a token of some real thing behind appearances; and I make it real by putting it into words. It is only by putting it into words that I make it whole; this wholeness means that it has lost its power to hurt me; it gives me, perhaps because by doing so I take away the pain, a great delight to put the severed parts together. Perhaps this is the strongest pleasure known to me. It is the rapture I get when in writing I seem to be discovering what belongs to what; making a scene come right; making a character come together. (p. 71)

From these intense, qualitative changes in perception, Woolf concludes that behind the cotton wool is hidden meaning:

We—I mean all human beings—are connected with this; that the whole world is a work of art; that we are parts of the work of art. Hamlet or a Beethoven quartet is the truth about this vast mass that we call the world. But there is no Shakespeare, there is no Beethoven; certainly and emphatically there is no God; we are the words; we are the music; we are the thing itself. And I see this when I have a shock. (p. 72)[4]

This sense of oceanic, expansive "oneness" with all around is a theme that appears again and again from those documenting different aspects of transient depersonalization and derealization experiences, not typically shared by those suffering from the clinical syndrome. In a sense, Amiel and Woolf are having opposite experiences, flip sides of the same coin. Woolf's blows of being and aliveness stand in stark contrast to Amiel's perpetual deadness and void. She describes breakthrough moments of peak connectedness with the world she's embedded in, true being. He, on the other hand, never connects with the world around him, and true being is replaced by reflection on what being might have been. She has blows and he has void.

Existentialism

The first encounter with depersonalization can be sudden and ferocious, a so-called *coup de vide* (blow of the void). Few literary works depict this more profoundly than the novel *Nausea*, by the French writer and philosopher Jean-Paul Sartre. Sartre is the giant in any discussion of existentialism, a philosophical theory that views human individuals as free and responsible agents able to willfully determine their actions. The term "existential angst" continues to figure in contemporary society, both as something of a cliché reminiscent of Woody Allen movies and as a genuine deep dread in the younger generations now contending with imminent and global threats to our planet.

As a philosophy with a positive message of ultimate human agency, existentialism can be thought of as a *counter* to depersonalization stemming from the alienation and dehumanization of the individual in the modern world. Interestingly, several existentialist writers depict depersonalization in their fictional characters so poignantly and realistically that one wonders if they themselves had experienced it, and whether it led them down a new and more enlightened path.

Sartre portrayed the misery of head-on encounters with pure depersonalization in his first, and arguably best, novel, *Nausea*.[5] Nothing in literature or in case histories quite equals this novel because, unlike Amiel's *Journal Intime*, it is not a written recording of feelings and thoughts, but rather experience as it happens. It is not a clinical overview, but rather the voice of depersonalization unfolding second by second in an individual's consciousness.

Nausea is the story of a French history student and writer, Antoine Roquentin, who is inexplicably horrified at his own existence. Told in an impressionistic style, using the device of a diary that has been unearthed, the story is within Roquentin, who interprets even mundane daily life in the provincial town of Bouville (Mudville) as unreal, or too real, and consequently nauseating. He even names the sickening sensations that build to a terrifying crescendo in his consciousness—"the filth."

"Things are bad!" the character Roquentin writes at one juncture. "Things are very bad: I have it, the filth, the Nausea. And this time it is new: it caught me in a café. Until now, cafés were my only refuge because they were full of people and well lighted: now there won't even be that anymore." Written in 1935, *Nausea* takes place in a far-removed time and place, yet Roquentin's hyperawareness and overanalyzing sounds very familiar to depersonalized individuals today, as exemplified by this chilling excerpt:

> I buy a newspaper along my way. Sensational news. Little Lucienne's body has been found. Smell of ink, the paper crumples between my fingers. The criminal has fled. The child was raped. They found her body, the fingers clawing at the mud. I roll the paper into a ball, my fingers clutching at the

paper; smell of ink; my God how strongly things exist today. Little Lucienne was raped. Strangled. Her body still exists, her flesh bleeding. She no longer exists. Her hands. She no longer exists. The houses. I walk between the houses, I am between the houses, on the pavement; the pavement under my feet exists, the houses close around me, as the water closes over me, on the paper the shape of a swan. I am. I am. I exist, I think, therefore I am; I am because I think, why do I think? I don't want to think any more, I am because I think that I don't want to be, I think that I . . . because . . . ugh! I flee. (p. 100)[5]

Princeton University lecturer Russell Nieli has written on the relationships between the works of William James, Martin Heidegger, and Jean-Paul Sartre and clinical depersonalization.[6] He explores how Heidegger expresses the derealization-depersonalization experience in terms of *dread* and *the Nothing*: "Dread is the beginning of the alienation process, the attentional disengagement from both self and world (ego and environment), and the gradual slipping away of both self and world into an all-encompassing anxious indifference." Heidegger sums it up as "unhomelike-and-uncanny" (*unheimlich*) (see Chapter 2).

In commenting on *Nausea*, Nieli writes:

While a mood of estrangement—of aloneness in one's own private world, of being cut off from the surrounding social and physical work—permeates the whole novel, what is designated by the term Nausea (and what is easily recognizable as acute attacks of the derealization-depersonalization experience) occur at definite, peak-instances. A gradual buildup in the feeling of estrangement precedes each attack: "I must finally realize that I am subject to these sudden transformations. The thing is that I rarely think: small metamorphoses accumulate in me without my noticing it, and then, one fine day, a veritable revolution takes place."

Precious little occurs in *Nausea* in terms of conventional plot. Roquentin's mind is the plot and reaches an important denouement late in the book. Wandering near a town beach, the protagonist sees through those things being enjoyed by everyone else and is filled with cynicism and disgust. Then, he boards the tram aimlessly and continues:

I lean my hand on the seat and pull it back hurriedly: it exists. This thing I'm sitting on, leaning my hand on is called a seat. They made it purposefully for people to sit on . . . I murmur: "It's a seat," a little like an exorcism. But the words stay on my lips: it refuses to go and put itself on the thing . . . It could just as well be a dead donkey . . . and I could be sitting on the donkey's belly, my feet dangling in the clear water. Things are divorced from their names. They are there, grotesque, headstrong, gigantic and it seems ridiculous to call them seats or say anything at all about them: I am in the midst of things, nameless things. Alone, without words, defenseless, they surround me, are beneath me, behind me, above me. They demand nothing, they don't impose themselves: they are there.

Roquentin's heady overconsciousness of objects and the names assigned to them builds with claustrophobic urgency until he plows past the conductor and jumps off the tram before it has time to stop. He finds himself in a park, where his phenomenological quest climaxes, in view of a massive chestnut tree. An all-important change finally occurs:

I drop onto a bench between great black tree trunks, between the black, knotty hands reaching towards the sky. A tree scrapes at the earth under my feet with a black nail. I would so like to let myself go, forget myself, sleep. But I can't, I'm suffocating: existence penetrates me everywhere, through the eyes, the nose, the mouth . . . And suddenly, suddenly, the view is torn away, I have understood, I have seen.

Later, he analyzes what has happened:

I can't say I feel relieved or satisfied; just the opposite, I am crushed. Only my goal is reached: I know what I wanted to know; I have understood all that has happened to me since January. The Nausea has not left me and I don't believe it will leave me soon; but I no longer have to bear it, it is no longer an illness or a passing fit: it is I . . . in the park just now. The roots of the chestnut tree were sunk in the ground just under my bench. I couldn't remember it was a root anymore. The words had vanished, and with them the significance of things . . . I was sitting, stooping forward, head bowed, alone in front of this black, knotty mass, entirely beastly, which frightened me. Then I had the vision. It left me breathless. Never, until these last few days, had I understood the meaning of existence.

Roquentin spends several pages formulating a theory about what has been revealed to him, and ultimately liberates him: the realization that existence is only in the moment, that everything else past or present or connected to a name is an illusion. Things exist and labels get in the way. For both Amiel and Roquentin, feeling unreal becomes a glimpse into a different, and in their eyes just as true, reality—momentary and timeless, not seen through the ordinary filters of the experiencing self. Amiel's perception includes infinite love of Deity, Roquentin's does not. But unlike Amiel, Roquentin refuses to let this glimpse behind the façade of life lock him in limbo, stuck between two worlds. Instead, he sees complete freedom and a call to action. By the end of *Nausea*, his manner of action becomes clear. He decides to devote his life to writing.

Clearly, Sartre himself followed that path, not by creating an introspective diary but rather by giving voice to the philosophy of existentialism. Basing his conception of self-consciousness loosely on Heidegger's thoughts on being, Sartre proceeds to sharply delineate intentional actions ("for themselves") from unintended ones ("in themselves"). It is a choice, he claims, to live one's life "authentically" and in a unified fashion, or not—this is the fundamental freedom of our lives.

While in *Nausea* the reader follows Roquentin throughout a process leading to a peak of depersonalization, the protagonist of Albert Camus' *The Stranger* is already existing within it.[7] There is no mystical unification with an infinite being, like Amiel's. Whereas for Sartre a sense of absurdness is inherent to human existence, for Camus absurdity had more to do with how one chooses to relate to the world. Published in 1942, *The Stranger* portrays the deadness of an unfeeling, robot-like existence. On first reading, students are often struck by the indifferent and blasé attitude of the character Mearsault, apparent in the very first lines of the novel: "Mother died today. Or, maybe, yesterday; I can't be sure. The telegram from the home says: YOUR MOTHER PASSED AWAY, FUNERAL TOMORROW, DEEP SYMPATHY. Which leaves the matter doubtful; it could have been yesterday."

In his study of depersonalization, Dugas described a patient much like Mearsault who "experienced a strong feeling of 'apathy' to the point that, according to him, had anything bad happened to his loved ones, he would only have felt unhappy in retrospect. Apathy can be so marked that patients will not struggle against any experience, however disturbing."[8] To a large degree, this defines Mearsault. Yet there is a philosophy behind his indifference. He lives in the moment without anxiety and worry, only a knowledge that human life is absurd and meaningless, but for the present moment in which to live. Again, describing a comparable patient many years earlier, Dugas writes that "he lives in the present. He is thus able to adapt to new situations and to feel at ease anywhere; his ongoing perceptions fully occupy his attention and he is not obsessed by memories or ruminations about the past."[8]

Written during World War II and the German occupation of France, Camus' message did not intend to illustrate pathology. It was, rather, a message of resistance to the reality tensions of the German occupation and, beyond that, a world that is largely indifferent. The only answer for the individual is to rebel against the absurdity and meaninglessness experienced by the mind. Accordingly, Mearsault is not passively indifferent, but rather actively avoidant, as a chosen life stance.

Set in Algiers, Mearsault kills an Arab in a spontaneous reaction to what's around him—the heat and glare of the sun. In the ensuing investigation and trial, he is convicted mainly for his failure to show "proper feelings" for his deceased mother, rather than for the crime of murder. Aghast at his apparent lack of love, the jury condemns him to death. As a literary work, the novel develops the concept of the absurd and the belief that a person can still be actively happy in the face of the absurd. For Mearsault, the apathy and numbness of depersonalization are reactions to the nature of human life itself—life's absurdity is driven home by the way in which he is tried and convicted. Happiness remains only in the moment, in the ways in which he adapts to his prison cell through a beam of sunshine coming into it, or from his ultimate moral victory over the blind mob awaiting his execution.

Spirituality in the Christian Tradition

The eradication of the individual self is a vital part of many spiritual traditions. Yet how this self-erasure is experienced by any individual is subject to the influences of the religions, cultures, and societies within which a person is embedded. The pathways to spiritual states of mind may vary greatly, yet all share Carl Jung's reflection: *who looks outside, dreams; who looks inside, awakes.* Many contemporary accounts of depersonalization have emerged in the form of memoirs that almost inevitably morph the traditions of Eastern and Western mystical traditions—something Amiel felt, but never formulated into doctrine. They include a flurry of accounts in the "Christian contemplative" tradition, as well as more secular works lacking any specific genre.

Contrary to popular assumptions, the Christian tradition goes beyond phenomena like St. Paul's being "blinded by the light." It also includes centuries-old mystical experiences involving the elimination of the individual self, in contrast to the personal, conversant relationship with Christ that fundamentalists espouse today. In the 1860s, the writings of the obscure Jesuit priest Jean-Pierre de Caussade were published, more than a century after they were written (he would certainly have been tried for heresy during his lifetime). Commenting on the no-self experiences, he wrote in 1731:

> Often indeed God places certain souls in this state, which is called emptiness of the spirit or of the intelligence; it is also called: being in nothingness (*etre dans le rien*). This annihilation of our own spirit disposes wonderfully to receive that of Jesus Christ. This mystical death of the operations of our own activity renders our soul apt for the reception of divine operations.[9]

Bernadette Roberts's *The Experience of No-Self*, published in 1993, reflects this type of being, and hearkens to Amiel's desire to be an "empty vessel" filled with the presence of God.[10] Roberts's book documents her personal struggle with mysterious moments of deep, silent "stillness" that from early childhood she interpreted as the presence of God. She entered a convent to further pursue the source of this stillness and, while reading in a garden, "felt an invisible film, or thin veil, come down over my head and shroud my mind . . . The first thing I noticed was that I could no longer see the words on the page; suddenly they had become characters without a meaning. I looked inward to encounter the usual obscure presence of God, but there was a gaping black hole where he had been. There arose from this center a pain so terrible, so enormous, I wondered how it could be contained."[11]

For nine months, Roberts writes, she experienced this intense feeling of pain and emptiness, but "then, from out of nothingness, this ash heap of misery, there gradually emerged a whole new life. . . . It was when God revealed himself as the stillpoint that I discovered my true existential union with Him." After nine years she left the convent, married, and raised four children. She wasn't disillusioned, but she wanted to see if this new state of mind was compatible with normal, day-to-day family life. The pervasive, periodic inner silences came and went, until while visiting a monastery near her home, she experienced "the silence" and awaited "the onset of fear to break it up." But "instead of the usual unlocalized center of myself, there was nothing there, it was empty; and at that moment of seeing this there was a flood of quiet joy, and I knew, finally I knew what was missing—it was my *self*" (p. 23).[11]

Predictably, the "joy of emptiness" began to wane. When she tried to regain it through meditation,

the empty space began to expand, and expanded so rapidly it seemed to explode; then, in the pit of my stomach I had the feeling of falling a hundred floors in a non-stop elevator, and in this fall every issue of life was drained from me. The moment of landing I knew: When there is no personal self, there is no personal God. . . . My mind could not comprehend what had happened; this event and everything that followed fell outside any frame of reference known to me . . . When I visually focused in on a flower, an animal, another person, or any particular object, slowly the particularity would recede into a nebulous Oneness, so that the object's distinctness was lost to my mind . . . it became impossible for the mind to perceive or retain any individuality when all visual objects either faded from the mind, gave way to something else, or were "seen through." (p. 36)[10]

Strikingly similar to Roquentin's awakening by the chestnut tree and Woolf's blows, this type of profoundly changed perception is hard to manage. For Roberts, intermittent terror returned with a vengeance: "The silence within was not seen as freedom from self; rather, it was seen as an imprisoned self, a frozen, immovable self that was all part of the scene, part of the insidious nothingness choking the life out of everything. Even now it had frozen my body on the spot. How could I survive another moment?" She drove to a downtown area for the comfort of crowds and activity: "Looking at the young people around me, I was glad they had a self; in fact, the greatest blessing I could wish upon all the peoples of the earth was to have a self" (p. 36).[11]

Roberts tried to resume a normal life again, while living with anticipatory anxiety over a recurrence of this new and unexpected fear. Then, while on a retreat, she made an effort to face it once and for all. Seeking to eliminate this demon through her usual meditative practices, the final experience is described much like an exorcism, or an orgasm:

My head grew hot, and all I could see were stars. My feet began to freeze. Finally I fell back against the hill in a convulsive condition with my heart beating wildly. . . . It took me a while to realize my body was lying still on the hill, because initially, I seemed not to have one. I knew a great change

had taken place. . . . God is neither the see-er or the seen, but the "seeing" . . .
After a long passage, the mind has finally come to rest, and rejoices in its
own understanding. . . . Now it was ready to take its rightful place in the immediacy and practicality of the now-moment. (p. 92)[10]

The View from the East

Undoubtedly, depersonalization and other dissociative experiences can be
shaped, influenced, and interpreted via existing religious and cultural biases.
What happens when someone from a purely secular background experiences
states of mind very similar to those of a religious person? Roquentin's encounter with the chestnut tree provides one answer. Suzanne Segal's *Collision
with the Infinite* provides another.

For many DDD sufferers, Segal's experiences hit close to home. Her book
centers on an event that occurred while boarding a bus in Paris in 1982. She
was 27 years old and pregnant. As a young woman Segal had been involved
with the Transcendental Meditation movement, which was particularly
trendy in the 1970s. After several years, however, she became disillusioned
and left the "madhouse that the organization had become." She then studied
at the University of California, Berkeley, where after two years she gained
a degree in English literature. She then moved to Paris, where she married
and gave birth to a daughter. As she waited in line to get on the Paris bus, a
life-altering event occurred. Suddenly she felt her ears pop, and was at once
"enclosed in a kind of bubble" that cut her off from the rest of the scene, and
left her acting and moving in the most mechanical way. In *Collision*, she
describes that moment in detail:

> I lifted my right foot to step up into the bus and collided head-on with an
> invisible force that entered my awareness like a silently exploding stick of
> dynamite, blowing the door of my usual consciousness open and off its
> hinges, splitting me in two. In the gaping space that appeared, what I had
> previously called "me" was forcefully pushed out of its usual location inside
> me into a new location that was approximately a foot behind and to the left
> of my head. "I" was now behind my body looking out at the world without
> using the body's eyes. (p. 55)[12]

Walking home from that bus ride, she felt like a "cloud of awareness"
was following her body. The cloud was a "witness" located behind her and

completely separate from body, mind, and emotions. The witness was constant and so was fear, the fear of complete physical dissolution. The next morning, when nothing had changed, she wondered if she was going insane, and if she would ever be herself again. What Segal referred to as the "witnessing" continued for months and her only relief came in sleep, into which she "plunged for as long and as often as possible." She explains, "In sleep, the mind finally stopped pumping out its unceasing litany of terror, and the witness was left to witness an unconscious mind."

Recalling her earlier experiences with Transcendental Meditation, it occurred to her that this might be some kind of "cosmic consciousness," something her guru had described to her as the first stage of "awakened awareness." But it seemed impossible to her that this hellish realm could have anything to do with an enlightened state. After months of the presence of this mystifying witness, it disappeared, Segal writes, leaving her in a new state that was far more baffling, and consequently more terrifying, than the experience of the preceding months: "The disappearance of the witness meant the disappearance of the last vestiges of the experience of personal identity. The witness had at least held a location for a 'me,' albeit a distant one. In the dissolution of the witness, there was literally no more experience of a 'me' at all. The experience of personal identity switched off and was never to appear again."

Although internally Segal knew that she had changed radically, no one else noticed. She functioned as smoothly as ever, "as if there were an unseen doer who acted perfectly." She even managed to earn a doctorate in psychology in the years to follow. And yet, she writes, "The oddest moments occurred when any reference was made to my name. If I had to write it on a check or sign it on a letter, I would stare at the letters on the paper and the mind would drown in perplexity. The name referred to no one. There was no Suzanne Segal anymore; perhaps there never had been" (p. 55).[12] She consulted psychiatrists in an attempt to understand what had happened to her. Some diagnosed her with depersonalization disorder. Others had no clear explanation. As she lived in this mysterious state day after day, she became increasingly filled with fear: "Everything seemed to be dissolving right in front of my eyes, constantly. Emptiness was everywhere, seeping through the pores of every face I gazed upon, flowing through the crevices of seemingly solid objects. The body, mind, speech, thoughts, and emotions were all empty; they had no ownership, no person behind them. I was utterly bereft of all my previous notions of reality."

She later reasoned that the fear that pervaded her life forever after the "bus hit" came from the mind's attempts to make sense of what had happened to her. She determined that the mind created fear because it had lost control of the illusion of the person Suzanne Segal. In time, a further shift occurred. Driving though a wintry landscape she observed that "everything seemed more fluid. The mountains, trees, rocks, birds, sky, were all losing their differences. As I gazed about, what I saw first was how they were one; then, as a second wave of perception, I saw the distinctions. From that day forth I have had the constant experience of both moving through and being made of the 'substance' of everything."

She contacted spiritual teachers within the California Buddhist community and gained reassurance, which helped ease the nonstop fear she had previously endured. She was also provided explanations in the form of Buddhist teachings regarding *anatta* (no-self) and *shunyata* (emptiness). Her kind of no-self experience was not only understood but actually being cultivated, through daily regimens of rituals and meditations, by those wanting to follow certain spiritual paths. Buddhism, she felt, provided a plausible explanation for it all. In simple terms, the Buddhist interpretation states that "personality functions" remain even when one's self has disappeared. These are known as *skandhas* or "aggregates," and include form, feelings, perceptions, thoughts, and consciousness. Their interaction creates the illusion of self, yet they do not actually make up the self—there is no self, Buddhism claims. When the truth of the *skandhas* is revealed, as suddenly happened to Segal at the bus stop, it is seen that there is no self, only the *skandhas* still functioning as they do. In Tibetan Buddhism this is known as the realization of *emptiness*, in Zen Buddhism as the realization of *no mind*.

Buddhism stresses that changes of consciousness are attained in stages: devotion (*saddha*), discipline (*sila*), detachment (*caga*), and depersonalization (*panna*). The rituals and self-preparation are essential lifelong processes, with depersonalization as the final goal. Understandably, an unplanned, unexpected fast-track to *panna* could be quite terrifying, even for someone with knowledge of Buddhism. When Segal's "collision" became widely known, she received numerous congratulations from spiritual teachers, both Eastern and Western. From India, the well-known guru Poonjaji wrote, "In between the arrival of the bus and your waiting to board, there was the Void where there was no past or future. This Void revealed itself to itself. This is a wonderful experience. It has to stay eternally with you. This is perfect freedom. You have become (moksha) of the realized sages."

Closer to home, one of Poonjaji's American-born disciples (who took the name Gangaji) reassured her: "This realization of the inherent

emptiness—which is pure consciousness—of all phenomena is true fulfillment. In the face of conditioned existence, much fear can be initially felt.
Ultimately, the fear is also revealed to be only that same empty consciousness." Unfortunately for Segal, the fear that had disappeared eventually
returned with renewed intensity, as happened to Bernadette Roberts. She
stopped all public appearances and withdrew into virtual seclusion. She continued meeting with fellow therapists and, in time, revealed that she had
suffered a long history of migraine headaches and, to the surprise of many,
she began to recover memories of abuse from her childhood. She died in
1997 of a brain tumor, before her revelations later in life and the impact of her
brain lesion could be further explored and understood.

Through a Glass, Darkly

Experiences of no-self can occur spontaneously, as in the cases and characters
described so far; they can also be induced, or facilitated, by mind-altering
drugs. Aldous Huxley's most famous work on the subject is *The Doors of
Perception*, published along with a second lengthy essay, *Heaven and Hell*,
in 1954.[13] Although his writings do not involve depersonalization as a disorder, *The Doors of Perception* describes the unreality and loss of the individual self through the use of psychedelics, specifically the cactus-derived
substance mescaline. Certain drugs can open the doors of the mind so that
different states of awareness can take hold, Huxley felt. Cultures around the
world used mescaline, peyote, psilocybin, or hashish for this very purpose in
their religious rites.

   In the presence of an investigator/companion and a tape recorder, Huxley
ingested mescaline and waited to record its effects, which were ultimately
recounted in *The Doors of Perception*. The onset of a new, different perception
began with a simple vase in the room that contained a rose, a carnation, and
an iris. He had noticed the colorful flowers earlier in the day, but now, under
the influence, he was not just looking at a flower arrangement: "I was seeing
what Adam had seen on the morning of his creation—the miracle, moment
by moment of naked existence. . . . I continued to look at the flowers, and in
their living light I seemed to detect the qualitative equivalent of breathing—
but of a breathing without returns to a starting point, with no recurrent ebbs
but only a repeated flow from beauty to heightened beauty, from deeper to
ever deeper meaning."

All the words Huxley had known from Buddhism—Mind, Suchness, the Void, the Godhead—now seemed completely understandable, he says, as reality was being experienced moment to moment by a "Blessed Not-I." Spatial relationships meant nothing while under mescaline. The mind was primarily concerned not with measures and locations, but with being and meaning. And along with indifference to space there went an even more complete indifference to time. Visually, what Huxley experienced took on a Van Gogh-like intensity. Secrets that were hidden, seen only as if "through a glass, but darkly," to use the biblical phrase, with the help of mescaline seemed not only clear and bright but also intensely detailed, as if the glass had become an electron microscope.

One 43-year-old writer who has experienced depersonalization chronically for more than 20 years has created his own metaphor to describe his feelings about higher consciousness: "To me depersonalization seems to have been my mind tapping at the door of some mystical experience, or even some kind of higher knowledge. But it never got in because it didn't know the password. So it walked away and decided it was just sick. The mind never knew what amazing things lay on the other side of that door, nor how to access them" (anonymous post on www.depersonalization.info). While Huxley could indeed articulate the ecstatic nature of his own self-induced experiences in compelling language, he was not so naïve to think that there could not also be a dark side to opening the doors of perception.

In *Heaven and Hell*, he brings up the point that visionary experience is not always pleasant. Hellish images and feelings can come from within or without as easily as sacred ones. "Sanity is a matter of degree," Huxley writes, "and for some, the universe can be transfigured—but for the worse. Everything in it, from the stars in the sky to the dust under their feet, is unspeakably sinister or disgusting; every event is charged with a hateful significance; every object manifests the presence of an In-swelling Horror, infinite, all-powerful, eternal" (p. 134).[13] Huxley pointed out that while blissful visions usually involve a pleasant sense of separation from the body, a "feeling of deindividualization" that is not disturbing, in more negative visionary experiences the body feels more dense and tightly packed. Unfortunately, "deindividualization" can often manifest itself as unpleasant. People subjected to it and experiencing persistent chronic depersonalization did not seek out a visionary experience or an opportunity to detach from their previous self. The result is much more hellish than heavenly, as evidenced by so many of today's personal accounts.

Alice in Wonderland

In the early 1950s, before writing *The Doors of Perception*, Huxley was trying his hand at screenwriting and living in the Santa Monica Canyon west of Los Angeles. This area was part of the literary L.A. scene at the time and hosted such full- or part-time residents as Huxley and his wife; novelists Christopher Isherwood, Charles Bukowski, Henry Miller, and Anaïs Nin; and the Beat poet Allen Ginsberg. Also living in the neighborhood was Ginsberg's cousin, a psychiatrist named Oscar Janiger. Janiger's primary interests as a doctor and scientist were the study of consciousness, the origins of creativity, and the mysterious nature of something he had experienced himself as a teenager in upstate New York—depersonalization.

It was inevitable that Janiger and Huxley would become acquainted before long, and they quickly learned that in addition to the obvious, they shared an interest in something else—a derivative from ergot, which, discovered by Albert Hofmann while working for the Swiss firm Sandoz Laboratories, came to be known as LSD-25. More than a decade before the drug made its way into popular culture amid Timothy Leary's mantra of "tune in, turn on, drop out," LSD was seen as possibly being a viable key to help unlock the doors of schizophrenia and other mental illnesses. Many people were interested in exploring its potential. But in 1954, Janiger began the first and largest comprehensive study of LSD, involving more than 950 adult volunteers from all walks of life, young and old alike. Like Huxley, Janiger was interested in tapping into those areas of the mind that might harbor untapped creative potential or provide glimpses into a broader reality than perceived in ordinary day-to-day life.

Participants were carefully screened for preexisting psychological problems and general health. The setting for their LSD session was a rented house with a small patio and garden. Objects in the room were limited to a few paintings, record albums, and assorted bric-a-brac. Another room was set up with art supplies for the purpose of a sub-study involving artists; for the hundred or so people who used this room, a colorful deer kachina doll served as a solitary model. Each participant was asked to write their impressions on small notecards and later give a full report of their experience; Janiger stayed nearby to monitor the experience but did not interfere with it. The artists were asked for two renderings of the kachina doll, one before LSD and one during.

Eight years later the study was completed; piles and piles of neatly stacked notecards, tapes, and all pertinent data remained in Janiger's files for nearly 40 years. A few minor scholarly papers reviewed some of the study's findings, but it wasn't long before LSD was a pariah, unobtainable legally, and a major drug of abuse within the 1960s counterculture and beyond. In the 1990s, however, new and unbiased interest in the positive uses of LSD began to enjoy a renaissance and continues to this day within mainstream psychiatry. Janiger passed away in 2001, but the complete record of his LSD experiments was published posthumously in 2003 in a book co-written with medical anthropologist Marlene Dobkin de Rios.[14] The published results of the study, which give detailed accounts of a broad spectrum of LSD-induced phenomena, bear relevance to the understanding of depersonalization:

> Of all the big changes you notice, the change in self-concept and body image is most immense. You feel at first no definite sharp location of yourself. This you, which stands outside yourself, shows no rigid shape. You feel dissociated and removed. Things, yourself, feel strange. You may have a strange reaction to the mirror, as if seeing a stranger. You feel able to step out of the rented costume of the self you held rigidly within narrow bounds. (p. 11)[14]

The recorded LSD experiences were more novel then, but are widely familiar today—visual disturbances, loss of time, vibrant colors, intensity of music, sense of oneness with the universe, and sensations of detachment and depersonalization. Condensed comments regarding depersonalization included: "I'm inside of me and outside of me at the same time . . . I seem to be able to watch myself like an observer . . . My voice has a detached quality . . . Funny things happen to your sense of ego. A sort of double personality permits me to be and at the same time to observe from the outside" (p. 55).[14] Interestingly, of the hundreds of volunteers, some of whom suffered anxiety, terror, and the fearful hallucinations that can accompany a "bad trip," none felt that the depersonalized or other dissociative aspects of the trip were difficult or unpleasant; they were transient, expected, and even pleasant. Furthermore, no cases of chronic depersonalization were reported after the fact as a result of the study.

Yet, for some DDD patients LSD triggered the condition; as with any mind-altering drug, many take it and only a fraction develop chronic depersonalization. Many factors likely affect outcome: the dosage and purity of the drug, the safeness of the physical setting and the presence or absence of others, and the fact that in Janiger's study participants were screened for mental wellbeing. For someone whose wellbeing is more fragile and tenuous, or who already has a propensity to dissociate, the "readiness" for a more positive drug-induced experience may not be there, and persistent depersonalization could be a risk and undesirable outcome.

An interesting finding of the study had to do with creativity, involving the artists' renditions of the kachina doll. Typically, the pre-LSD renderings were realistic, predictable, and drawn to scale, and reflected an artist's known style. The LSD-inspired paintings and drawings were brighter, more abstract, less representational, and more emotionally compelling. Some of the artists reported that it was as if for the first time they had been freed up of all the learned ways, the repetitive ruts, and the baggage to which they had become accustomed in daily life. They were able to fuse with the object being perceived and represented, and understood what Picasso meant by "When you paint an apple, you should be an apple."

In the mid-1950s, the young British writer Colin Wilson wrote a book called *The Outsider*, which examined the lives and work of certain people who made a lasting impact on their respective creative fields. It also peered into the psyches of the fictional characters created by these people. From Dostoevsky to Camus to Tolstoy to Nietzsche to the Russian dancer Nijinsky, the subjects of *The Outsider* all share an inherent detachment from day-to-day reality. "The Outsider is not sure who he is," Wilson states. "He has found an 'I' but it is not his true 'I.' His main business is to find his way back to himself" (159).[15]

This, in fact, is one of the dilemmas sometimes facing those with chronic depersonalization: "If I feel as if I have lost my old self and am filled with fear because the world seems strange, where is my new self?" A philosopher or artist might argue that there is potential for a transformational transition to a more liberated and enlightened, "new" self. A mental health professional would say that the "old" self was more troubled than its surface suggested or revealed, and that a "new" self inevitably involves knowing, reworking, and healing the "old" one. And the two views are not incompatible.

Back from the Looking Glass

In 2001, Andrew Newberg of the Department of Radiology at the University of Pennsylvania Medical Center published two single-photon emission computerized tomography (SPECT) studies, one looking at Franciscan nuns and the other at Tibetan Buddhist meditators.[16] In both groups, intense meditation was associated with increased brain activity in the prefrontal cortex, the dorsolateral and medial orbitofrontal, and the cingulate gyrus—areas involved in cognitive control and focused concentration on the self. Moreover, there was a relative shutdown of the prefrontal cortex, which is involved in executing processing and planning, and an overactivation of the superior parietal lobe, reflecting the altered sense of being, mind, body, and space experienced during meditation. As discussed in the previous chapter, similar areas are involved in the experience of depersonalization.

Newberg has studied brain activity and meditation for two decades now and is a founding father of the emerging field of neurotheology. His research group has scanned people's brains as they perform practices from diverse traditions, from various forms of meditation and prayer to speaking in tongues and entering trance states. Survey studies have included detailed descriptions of experiences from a variety of spiritual traditions. Five elements have emerged as common across many enlightenment experiences:[17]

- *Intensity*: Enlightenment experiences are commonly considered to be the most intense experiences that a person has ever had, often associated with feelings like love, joy, and awe. The intensity is likely associated with activation of the limbic system, the brain's primary emotional center.
- *A sense of oneness or unity*: During the experience, the person feels a profound sense of connectedness with the rest of humanity, God, or the Universe, associated with a decrease of activity in the parietal lobe, responsible for integrating sensory information and creating a spatial representation of the self.
- *A sense of clarity*: People feel as if a veil has been lifted and that they are now seeing and understanding the world in ways they never have before. This sense of clarity and new-found insightfulness is associated with the thalamus, a brain structure central to integration and consciousness.
- *A sense of surrender*: Most people describe enlightenment experiences as *happening to them* rather than as something that they made happen, a "going along for the ride," associated with frontal lobe deactivation and a loosening of purposeful control.

- *Transformation:* Various aspects of one's life can change through transformative experiences, including mental wellbeing, physical wellbeing, meaning and purpose, and spirituality. Brain scan studies have documented differences in the brains of long-time meditators compared with non-meditators, with the former exhibiting increased activity and thickness in the frontal lobes, which may subsume the solidification of enlightenment experiences over time, on the gradual path to transformation.

Nonetheless, the issue of how the practices in question might affect people with chronic depersonalization has not been explored in Newberg's studies, or elsewhere, and so remains unanswered. Anecdotally, we do know that some develop incrementally unpleasant depersonalization experiences during meditation practices and come to abandon them. We also know that many with DDD benefit from deep breathing, meditation, and meditative yoga supplementation to their treatments, often recommended by clinicians. Every person is different, and has only explored limited paths to healing. Undoubtedly, learning to be more mindful, and present in the now, holds healing potential for most.

Depersonalization-like experiences appear in many creative works, with many interpretations throughout the centuries. That will continue, often through venues like literary quarterlies, or the internet, where everyone can articulate their impressions of a baffling and isolating condition through graphics, poetry, or prose. We offer the following poem, by Cheswayo Mphanza, as an example.

Frame Six

These days I wake in the used light of someone's spent life.
I am often a stranger to myself;
I have no place of origin—no home.
I keep remembering everything in two time zones at once.
Who knows, maybe I myself am called something else than myself.
Not so much a name, but the result of a name.
It's a strange sensation to yell out: *this is me!*
In every place I've watched caravans of sorrow—

I run like all the other men, chasing my shadow down alleys.
            Sometimes in the spaces, there is fear—
my mind deepens into them.
            From calm to fear my mind moves, then *moves*—
            in light part nightmare and part vision fleeing.
The voice rises on a storm of grackles, then returns—half elegy, half serenade.[18]

10

Biological Treatments

We should make it clear that getting help isn't a sign of weakness—it's a sign of strength.

—Michelle Obama

The world of depersonalization, like the ocean, is vast, mysterious, and deep. But someone who is drowning couldn't care less about that: they want to be safely back in the boat or on shore. People suffering from depersonalization/derealization disorder (DDD) make an appointment to see a psychiatrist because they are in pain. Some want and expect relief from that pain just as if it were the result of a broken limb or an infection. Others are more content to find hope, a piece of buoyant debris to cling to while awaiting rescue. Unfortunately, they sometimes visit doctor after doctor, finding neither. Even when they are lucky enough to locate a psychiatrist who is familiar with their disorder, there is no simple treatment, no magic bullet to make that pain go away quickly, no miraculous rescue. But relief can be found as one embarks on the journey toward complete recovery. Physicians have at their disposal a large arsenal of pharmaceutical treatments with which to combat mental illness. Not all medicines affect everyone the same way, but the medicines in use today are quite sophisticated and offer a promising rainbow of possibilities.

The past two decades have witnessed an expansion and refinement of medication treatment options for the disorder. Though there are no medications for DDD that are officially approved by the U.S. Food and Drug Administration, we now know that a number of different medication classes can be used, and often have positive results. Historically, DDD was considered a disorder notoriously resistant to medication treatment, but this perspective has gradually shifted. Pharmacological treatment trials, though still few compared to many other psychiatric disorders, have proliferated and yielded promising outcomes.

Feeling Unreal. Second Edition. Daphne Simeon and Jeffrey Abugel, Oxford University Press. © Oxford University Press 2023. DOI: 10.1093/oso/9780197622445.003.0010

The history of the medicines used, and often cited as being effective for treating depersonalization/derealization (dpdr), is as old as the study of the disorder itself. In 1939, Paul Schilder reported favorable results in nine patients with severe depersonalization using the central-nervous-system stimulant metrazol (pentamethylenetetrazol).[1] Others reported success with methamphetamine,[2] thiopental,[3] D-amphetamine and amobarbital.[4,5] These drugs are rarely used today, because of their significant risks and the availability of safer alternatives; however, in the past, stimulants and barbiturates were prominent in the limited pharmacological armamentarium for psychiatric disorders.

Electroconvulsive therapy (ECT), recommended in some of the earliest papers discussing depersonalization treatment, was ultimately found to be more effective for depression alone. Fifty years ago, a study of 15 patients with severe depression and depersonalization reported that while depression improved following ECT, depersonalization did not.[6] In a contemporary cohort of 117 patients with DDD, three had received ECT treatment: two had experienced no change in dpdr symptoms, and one had markedly worsened.[7]

In the 1950s, the first effective modern pharmacotherapy for major depression emerged quite by accident. Developed as a treatment for tuberculosis, monoamine oxidase inhibitors (MAOIs) turned out to be much more successful in elevating mood. To this day, they are still prescribed as potent antidepressants, usually when a patient has not responded to other classes of antidepressants available today. This class of drugs was followed, in Europe and in the United States, by the tricyclic antidepressants (TCAs). Like the MAOIs they were effective against depression and panic disorder but had fewer risks or side effects. Although a few reports have appeared about isolated individuals with DDD who benefit from these medications, the overall impression remains that for most part, while they may help combat anxiety, panic, and depression, they do little for dpdr directly.

What medications, then, can be used to treat DDD, and what is the evidence?

Retrospective Treatment Report from 117 DDD Patients

In the series of 117 patients with DDD studied by the New York group, participants were asked to describe all the treatments that they had previously received.[7] If a medication "trial" appeared reasonable enough in dose and in duration to count as an "adequate" treatment trial, it was tallied into the totals. This retrospective record revealed that there was limited success, spanning a variety of different medications, in treating DDD, though it is important to be aware of potential bias inherent in such a study: any DDD sufferer with sustained symptom improvement would likely not have met the diagnostic criteria for study participation. Participants were asked whether each medication had left their dpdr the same or worse; slightly better; or definitely better. The information gathered was based on patients' best memory, often from a long time before. Therefore, the findings are not as reliable as conducting an actual treatment trial, where investigators strictly record the numbers of weeks of treatment, the maximum dose reached, and compliance with taking the medication, and do repeated symptom ratings.

The study reported no "efficacy" (the medical term for effectiveness) for the traditional TCAs. Out of a total of 31 treatment trials, only two had led to slight improvement and one to definite improvement. As already stated, the TCAs are an older medication class that includes nortriptyline (Pamelor), imipramine (Tofranil), desipramine (Norpramin), amitriptyline (Elavil), and clomipramine (Anafranil). They are effective and inexpensive antidepressants and anxiolytics, but often have more side effects than the newer antidepressants and anxiolytics that we will be discussing shortly.

Like the TCAs, the older MAOIs appeared equally ineffective. Of a total of 16 reported trials, only two had resulted in slight improvement. As stated earlier, nowadays MAOIs are generally prescribed to treat refractory depression that has not responded to other classes of antidepressants. Monoamine oxidase is an enzyme that breaks down "monoamines" in the brain. By inhibiting monoamine oxidase, MAOIs extend the life of these amines. The MAOIs have a broad scope of action, affecting the levels of serotonin, norepinephrine, and dopamine in the brain. Taking high doses of MAOIs can sometimes be helpful in stimulating more alertness, similar to amphetamines. The MAOIs include phenelzine (Nardil), tranylcypromine (Parnate), isocarboxazid (Marplan), and the newer selegiline patch (Emsam). Although these drugs have proven very effective for depression and anxiety, doctors don't prescribe them frequently because serious interactions with medications, and with foods containing a lot of tyramine, can occur.

Another antidepressant, bupropion (Wellbutrin, Zyban), known to work for depression as well as for smoking cessation, was similarly ineffective in DDD. Of 11 individuals who had tried it, only one reported having experienced definite improvement. Similarly, the antidepressant venlafaxine (Effexor) appeared ineffective; of seven trials, none had resulted in improvement. Venlafaxine belongs to the serotonin and norepinephrine reuptake inhibitor (SNRI) class of antidepressants, which effectively lead to an increase of both serotonin and norepinephrine activity in the brain.

The 117 participants reported a total of 60 selective serotonin reuptake inhibitor (SSRI) trials. This commonly prescribed class of medications is, currently, the "first line" treatment for depression, anxiety, and obsessive-compulsive disorder. SSRIs were designed to act on specific neurotransmitter systems, unlike many older drugs that impact multiple neurotransmitter systems at once. They affect how much serotonin is available in the brain by blocking its reabsorption during transmission from one nerve cell in the brain to another; it is this blocking action that causes an increased amount of serotonin to become available to the next nerve cell. Serotonin is thought to be involved in depression, anxiety, as well as obsessive-compulsive spectrum conditions. In addition to fluoxetine (Prozac), this class of medications includes sertraline (Zoloft), paroxetine (Paxil), fluvoxamine (Luvox), citalopram (Celexa), and escitalopram (Lexapro). Of the 60 SSRI trials reported in the study, 14 had led to slight improvement and nine to definite improvement of dpdr symptoms, according to the participants. This 38% effectiveness appeared promising for a retrospective report, certainly better than that of the other antidepressants—we'll examine more rigorous research of the SSRIs in treating DDD shortly.

Other medications can be used to treat anxiety, but not depression. Benzodiazepines are central nervous system depressants (medicines that dampen excitation and slow down the nervous system) and include alprazolam (Xanax), clonazepam (Klonopin), lorazepam (Ativan), and many others. They can be used to treat a variety of anxiety disorders such as generalized anxiety, social anxiety, and panic as well as anxiety of any origin. Dependence and tolerance to these medications develops after taking them on a regular basis for several weeks, so a person can become addicted if not using them judiciously, or may experience withdrawal symptoms if the dose is decreased too rapidly or the medication is suddenly stopped. Benzodiazepines enhance the action of the neurotransmitter gamma amino butyric acid (GABA). Once released, neurotransmitters signal inhibition or excitation of neighboring brain cells; GABA is the major inhibitory neurotransmitter in our brain. The function of GABA is to slow and calm things down. Benzodiazepines increase the action of GABA, thus promoting inhibition or calming.

Thirty-five benzodiazepine trials were reported by the 117 DDD participants. Of these, eight (23%) led to slight improvement and 10 (29%) led to definite improvement; in other words, about half of patients had benefited from taking them. Again, this appeared to be quite a promising response for a condition considered hard to treat. To this day, there are no clinical trials that have examined the effectiveness of benzodiazepines in DDD, in large part because these are not ideal medications to be taking regularly unless necessary, and in combination with other medications that are not addictive. Undoubtedly, though, they seem to work at least partly for some patients, usually the highly anxious ones. By significantly diminishing anxiety, they can result in some improvement of dpdr symptoms, especially when the latter are significantly anxiety-driven.

Another anti-anxiety medication, with an entirely different action from the benzodiazepines, is buspirone (Buspar), which acts as an antagonist of the serotonin 5HT 1A receptor. Of the 15 trials of buspirone reported in the 117 participants, none were efficacious.

Nine stimulant medication trials were reported in the study, and two of these had led to slight improvement. These medications enhance the dopamine system in the brain, and are used to treat conditions such as attention-deficit disorder, because they improve attention and focusing. Like benzodiazepines, they have the potential for addiction.

Of the remaining classes of medications reported in the study, all were virtually ineffective. These included mood-stabilizing medications such as lithium (none of nine trials worked) and anticonvulsants such as valproic acid (only one of 12 trials led to slight improvement). It is very important to note, however, that at the time this study was conducted, the anticonvulsant and mood stabilizer lamotrigine (Lamictal) was not on the psychiatric horizon.

Importantly, antipsychotic medications, typically used to treat psychotic disorders such as schizophrenia, appeared to do nothing for dpdr, even though these were commonly prescribed for depersonalization in the past, in part because some viewed DDD as a psychosis. In fact, antipsychotics are still used in general psychiatric practice as a *primary* treatment for DDD. None of the 13 trials of the older "conventional" antipsychotics, and none of the seven trials of the newer "atypical" antipsychotics, exhibited efficacy in treating dpdr.

Do SSRIs Work for DDD?

In the early 1990s, a small open series[8] and two single case reports[9,10] had suggested that SSRIs alone may be effective in treating DDD. It was thought that these might work because of their efficacy in treating obsessive-compulsive spectrum disorders; obsessional thinking and ritualistic checking are often, but not invariably, part of the clinical picture of DDD. In 2004, a definitive treatment study was published in the *British Journal of Psychiatry* examining the efficacy of fluoxetine (Prozac) in DDD.[11] In this study, 25 individuals with DDD were randomly assigned to fluoxetine treatment and 25 to placebo treatment. The patients were not allowed to be taking any other medications. The treatment lasted 10 weeks, and participants built up to a rather high dose of fluoxetine, on average about 50 mg/day. The study reported that the individuals taking fluoxetine showed significant *overall* improvement in their dpdr symptoms compared to those taking placebo. When this improvement was "corrected" for changes in anxiety and depression, fluoxetine no longer appeared better than placebo. This raised the question of whether changes in dpdr symptoms might not have been primary, but rather secondarily mediated by lessened depressive or anxiety symptoms that were fueling the dpdr. Bottom line, however, improvement is improvement no matter the reasons.

The average overall improvement in dpdr symptoms with fluoxetine in this clinical trial was rated as "minimal," suggesting that though the improvement was statistically significant compared to placebo, and clinically worthwhile for some of the patients, it was not for others. A common subjective report by participants who later turned out to have taken fluoxetine, when the study "blind" was broken, was that their depersonalization symptoms had not really changed, but rather they felt better and were less bothered by them. It can be difficult to know how to interpret such a statement, not infrequently encountered in clinical treatments. Notably, the DDD sufferers who derived the greatest benefit from fluoxetine were those who had a comorbid anxiety disorder that also improved with the medication. No further SSRI clinical trials in DDD have been conducted since the original one. The broad conclusion is that SSRIs are always worth trying in DDD, and have some efficacy. But the outcome varies, and in part depends on the presence of other symptoms that are SSRI-responsive.

Clomipramine: An Older Serotonergic Medication

Clomipramine (Anafranil) is a TCA that, like the later SSRIs, treats depression, panic, and obsessive-compulsive disorder. Like other TCAs, clomipramine inhibits norepinephrine and serotonin reuptake, thereby increasing their concentration at receptor sites. However, in contrast to most other TCAs, clomipramine is a very potent serotonin reuptake inhibitor—like the SSRIs. It is this ability to alter serotonin activity that makes it effective in treating OCD like the SSRIs do, but unlike other TCAs. Clomipramine also has a mild sedative effect, due to its anticholinergic properties, which may be helpful in alleviating anxiety and facilitating sleep.

In 1998, Simeon and colleagues published a preliminary study examining clomipramine versus desipramine in the treatment of DDD (desipramine is another TCA that does not have strong serotonergic properties like clomipramine).[12] Unfortunately, the small numbers in the study did not allow statistical comparison of the two medications. However, of the four participants who were treated with clomipramine and did not discontinue treatment early on, two experienced significant improvement of their dpdr symptoms. One of these two patients showed almost complete remission for years afterward while continuing to take clomipramine, yet suffered setbacks whenever he attempted to discontinue clomipramine or switch over to other similar medications like SSRIs. This older medication still merits consideration in treating DDD, especially in patients who cannot tolerate SSRIs either due to general side effects, or because the "numbing" that is sometimes induced by SSRIs contributes to a heightened sense of depersonalization.

Lamotrigine: The New Hope

After the emergence of SSRIs, a flurry of interest in treating DDD with lamotrigine began to surface. This interest unfolded from a report in the *Archives of General Psychiatry* in 2000.[13] Although NMDA antagonists like ketamine induce potent dissociation by increasing glutamate transmission at non-NMDA glutamate receptors, it was found that pretreatment of healthy volunteers with lamotrigine, which inhibits glutamate release, lessened ketamine-induced dissociation. The finding gave hope that treatment with lamotrigine might be helpful in dissociative conditions.

A promising short report of lamotrigine treatment was published in 2001.[14] Eleven DDD patients who had proved resistant to previous medication treatments, all but one still taking SSRIs, were treated with lamotrigine. Since lamotrigine is a known treatment of mood disorders, it is important to note than none of these patients had mood symptoms at the time of the treatment. It turned out that six of the 11 patients experienced dpdr symptom improvement, ranging from 40% to 80%, at lamotrigine daily doses of 200 mg to 250 mg. However, these patients were not partaking in a methodical and placebo-controlled treatment study. They were random individuals who had not responded to other medications (mainly SSRIs), and so lamotrigine had been added to their medication regimen.

Subsequently, the same researchers embarked on a systematic study of lamotrigine in DDD, published in 2003.[15] They conducted what is known as a "crossover" treatment trial, a design in which all participants received both lamotrigine and placebo, in random order. Nine patients participated in this study and, disappointingly, it was completely negative—none of the nine showed any notable improvement while taking lamotrigine.[15] In fact, there was not even a placebo response in this small study, a rather unusual happening in any treatment trial. The authors speculated that this treatment failure might have been due, at least in part, to the fact that most of these DDD patients had had very chronic and refractory dpdr since childhood, and it is generally thought that patients with a very long illness duration tend to be less medication-responsive.

Regardless, later studies with lamotrigine have proved more hopeful. In 2006, the same British group published a treatment trial examining lamotrigine as an "add-on" treatment for DDD.[16] The study included 32 patients, most of whom were already taking SSRIs, SNRIs, or TCAs. Over half (56%) showed at least 30% symptom improvement with the addition of lamotrigine. This was not a rigorous controlled clinical trial, but rather a "naturalistic" open-ended treatment for six months to almost two years. The final dose was as high as 600 mg daily. It turned out that, overall, higher lamotrigine dosages resulted in greater symptom improvement, highlighting the importance of maximizing lamotrigine dosage, as tolerated, if response is not adequate at lower dosages. The dosage increase can be monitored by obtaining lamotrigine peak and trough blood levels. It also turned out that those with the most severe initial symptoms showed the greatest improvement. The investigators speculated that both serotonergic and glutamatergic mechanisms may be at play in DDD, and that medication interventions might therefore be more successful when targeting both neurotransmitters. But is this the case?

Though we do not have a definitive answer on the benefit of combining SSRIs and lamotrigine, the largest lamotrigine clinical trial to date was published in 2011, and now stands as the definitive study supporting the effectiveness of lamotrigine, in and of itself, in treating DDD.[17] The study enrolled 80 men with DDD who were not taking any medications; half received lamotrigine and half placebo. Of the 36 patients who adhered to the 12-week lamotrigine treatment, 26 (72%) were deemed to be responders, defined as least 50% reduction in dpdr symptoms. On average, the lamotrigine-treated group experienced a marked 46% reduction in symptoms as measured by the Cambridge Depersonalization Scale. On the other hand, only 16% of those who received placebo were responders. Patients were treated with a daily dose of up to 300 mg, reached by the eighth week of treatment, giving the medication a further full month to "kick in." This study is, presently, the last report on lamotrigine treatment in the DDD literature. Here we should note that though this article was "retracted" three years later by the journal's editors for using extensive wording from another publication without quotation marks, the data were not questioned.

Opioid Receptor Antagonists

Opioid receptor antagonists continue to be of interest in the treatment of dissociation generally, and DDD specifically. In Chapter 8 we provided some relevant background regarding the brain's endogenous opioid systems. Naltrexone is a nonspecific opioid receptor antagonist that at low dosages blocks the mu opioid receptors (the receptors involved in pain and mediating analgesia). At much higher doses, naltrexone also blocks other opioid receptors—blockade of the kappa opioid receptors might be of particular interest here, as the kappa opioid agonist enadoline has been found to induce a "pure" depersonalization syndrome in healthy volunteers (see Chapter 8).

Naltrexone at a high dose of 200 mg/day was reported to decrease general dissociative symptoms in patients with borderline personality disorder over a two-week treatment period.[18] Nalmefene, a medication like naltrexone that is not marketed in the United States, was reported to decrease emotional numbing in eight veterans with posttraumatic stress disorder.[19] What about dpdr more specifically? Nuller and colleagues[20] reported results from an intravenous naloxone trial in 11 patients with chronic DDD. Naloxone is a medication very similar to naltrexone but much shorter-acting; it is administered only intravenously. Of the 11 patients, three experienced complete remission and seven had marked improvement in depersonalization symptoms with treatment. However, this study reported only immediate treatment results after a single intravenous dose, leaving many questions unanswered.

Dr. Simeon's group published a DDD naltrexone treatment study in 2005.[21] Fourteen participants were treated with the medication for six to 10 weeks in what is known as an "open" treatment trial (one without a placebo control). The average naltrexone dose was fairly high, at 120 mg/day, aimed at blocking opioid receptors as broadly as possible. Three patients were rated as "very much improved" by the end of the treatment, and another one as "much improved." On average, dpdr symptoms decreased by about 30% across all participants.

Interestingly, in 2015 a German publication reported on the use of very-low-dose naltrexone for treating dissociation, at dosages of 2 to 6 mg/day, though not in DDD.[22] Of the 15 patients with "severe trauma-related and dissociative disorders," 11 were reported to have experienced an immediate positive effect and seven claimed lasting help.

Taken together, naltrexone and other opioid receptor antagonists are reasonable medications to consider in treating dpdr, supported by some evidence, though dosing guidelines are murky. Pure kappa opioid receptor antagonists, which may be of interest in dpdr as discussed earlier in this section, have been in the development pipeline for years now but have not reached the market. The marketed controlled medication buprenorphine is a *mixed* mu receptor agonist and kappa receptor antagonist. Though there are no reports of its use in treating DDD, *elevated* dissociation scores have been reported in patients taking buprenorphine for the treatment of opioid use disorder.[23]

Other Medications

Other medication options for people with DDD are more experimental, in the sense that they have not been the subject of any research study. Undoubtedly, some individuals benefit from benzodiazepine treatment (e.g., clonazepam). As described in the cohort of 117 DDD participants, about half reported having derived some benefit. This is particularly true in those who also experience strong anxiety or panic, which typically exacerbates their dpdr. However, others report that while benzodiazepines may have lessened their anxiety, these medications did not impact symptoms of dissociation at all, or even made them feel more spacy and absent. Regardless, benzodiazepines have the potential for tolerance and abuse, and should be used as adjuvants, not as first-line treatment. They are typically most helpful early in the course of DDD, or during exacerbations, when they can be taken on an "as-needed" (prn) basis rather than as a standing dose. Taken judiciously when a patient experiences peaks in symptom intensity, they can break the cycle of mounting anxiety and depersonalization.

Some DDD patients find that stimulant medications help them focus in the midst of the dpdr fog, and they may feel more clear-headed and present. The improvement appears to be rather minor, but for selected patients, especially those with pronounced subjective cognitive difficulties, stimulants can have a positive effect. There is also some theoretical rationale for using medications that enhance dopamine in depersonalization. Dopamine DA1 receptors enhance sensory input to the amygdala, one of the emotional centers of the brain. Another group of dopamine receptors, known as DA2 receptors, decrease the inhibition of the amygdala by the prefrontal cortex. Therefore, increased activity at either of these two dopamine receptors might be expected to enhance emotional activation in the brain. This is relevant since, as we discussed in Chapter 8, neurobiological models of depersonalization include diminished limbic reactivity.

A variety of stimulant medications are available, such as dextroamphetamine (Dexedrine), methylphenidate (short-acting Ritalin and longer-acting variants), amphetamine/dextroamphetamine salts (Adderall and Adderall Extended Release), and lisdexamfetamine (Vyvanse). As with benzodiazepines, stimulants are controlled substances with the potential for abuse and dependence and should be prescribed with caution and careful monitoring of their effectiveness. DDD patients who experience a lot of anxiety may feel worse when they take a stimulant. Like benzodiazepines, stimulants are useful when taken as needed, for example when a patient is feeling strongly depersonalized and has a challenging workload. Before taking a stimulant, it is always worth trying nonstimulant medications with stimulating properties, such as the dopaminergic antidepressant bupropion, which some patients with DDD find helpful.

Another class of medications of interest in treating DDD, again not systematically studied, are medications that modulate the noradrenergic system. Norepinephrine (noradrenaline) is one of the neurotransmitters in the brain that plays an important role in enhancing attention and alertness, as well as encoding emotional information, and there exists some biological evidence for noradrenergic dysregulation and sympathetic nervous system involvement in DDD (Chapter 8), as well as for early attentional processing difficulties under demanding conditions (Chapter 7). One example of such a medication is atomoxetine (Strattera), a noradrenergic reuptake inhibitor marketed for the treatment of attention-deficit/hyperactivity disorder (ADHD). Another class of noradrenergic medications are known are alpha-agonists and include clonidine and guanfacine. Like stimulants, these medications have the potential to increase anxiety in some with DDD, though others may feel less anxious, so anxiety needs to be monitored during a treatment trial.

As we discussed, antipsychotics are generally not helpful in DDD, and make many patients feel worse. However, there are occasional patients who have severely anxiety-evoking and destabilizing dpdr, or are prone to extreme cognitive elaborations and distortions of their dpdr experiences, who may benefit from very low dosages of atypical antipsychotics such as risperidone (Risperdal) or aripiprazole (Abilify). A trial of these medications may be worthwhile in those who have partly benefited from SSRIs but have not had an adequate response. An alternative medication for DDD patients who become severely anxious and depersonalized in a variety of situations, or when emotionally dysregulated, is the beta-blocker propranolol, used on an as-needed or standing basis.

Altogether, then, of our currently available medications, some have been shown to have an anti-depersonalization effect, with SSRIs and lamotrigine being the most substantiated. Other medications can be used to combat DDD's gamut of symptoms, from high anxiety and panic to low mood, difficulties with attention, mind-emptiness, hyperawareness, numbing, emotional dysregulation, and obsessive ruminations. Whether they work on dpdr more directly or more indirectly, by ameliorating other symptoms that fuel the dissociation, they are all worth considering in treatment.

Working with your Psychiatrist

The pharmacological treatment of DDD begins with the more standard medication approaches. If the response to SSRIs (and related medications such as

SNRIs and clomipramine) and/or lamotrigine is inadequate, a more "trial-and-error" (judicious and well-monitored) approach with various other medications that make some "clinical sense" is the current state of the art. Clearly, treating depersonalization pharmaceutically is still partly evidence-based and partly good-sense alchemy, and the medications currently available to us are often not as effective as we would like them to be. Had DDD been given the scientific and clinical attention that many other psychiatric disorders have received over the years, maybe this would not be the case. Hopefully, the future holds promise for expanding the medication armamentarium for DDD, now that the condition has captured more mainstream traction during the past two decades, and with new psychotropic medications reaching the market with some regularity.

Transcranial Magnetic Stimulation

A newer and promising non-medication treatment for DDD is repetitive transcranial magnetic stimulation (TMS). TMS is a noninvasive brain stimulation treatment technique that induces a magnetic field on the scalp, able to penetrate the brain within a limited target area and altering neuronal excitation in the targeted region. Low-frequency protocols decrease cortical excitability, whereas high-frequency protocols increase neuron excitability in the targeted area. TMS is now known to be effective for treating a variety of psychiatric disorders such as depression and obsessive-compulsive disorder. Two promising studies have begun the investigation of TMS effectiveness in DDD. Two brain regions have so far been examined as targets, the temporoparietal junction (TPJ) and the ventral prefrontal cortex (VPC).

As we discussed in Chapter 8, the TPJ was first established as a brain region of great interest in DDD following the *American Journal of Psychiatry* publication in 2000 by Simeon and colleagues from Mount Sinai, New York. The study described altered brain activity in DDD in this key brain region, which is seminal to multisensory integration, visuospatial perspective, self-processing, self/other distinction, and embodiment—all crucial to an intact sense of self. Based on this positron emission tomography (PET) imaging finding, Dr. Mantovani of Columbia University, in collaboration with Dr. Simeon, conducted the first TMS treatment study in DDD, published in 2011.[24] Twelve participants received three weeks of TMS (five sessions per week) to the right TPJ. The majority were medicated, but there had been no medication adjustments for at least two months. Two patients also had major depression, and four had anxiety disorders. At the conclusion of the three weeks, six of the 12 participants were classified as responders, defined as at least 50% symptom reduction: four were full responders and two were partial responders, with an average symptom decrease on the Cambridge Depersonalization Scale of 49%. Five of these six responders entered a second treatment phase that consisted of another three weeks of TMS to the same region, in order to examine further improvement; symptoms declined by another 15% from the pretreatment baseline. Notably, neither depression nor anxiety scores significantly decreased during the TMS treatment. A later analysis of the data revealed that the magnitude of the TMS response was specifically correlated with the symptom score for anomalous body experiences, as would be expected for this brain region.[25]

In 2014, the London research group published a study examining the effect of TMS on dpdr symptoms.[26] Two brain regions were targeted: the right TPJ (as in the earlier study above), associated with dpdr sensory alterations, and the right ventrolateral prefrontal cortex (VLPFC), implicated in dpdr hypoemotionality. A single TMS treatment session was delivered in this pilot exploration. Seventeen DDD patients were randomized to receive treatment to one of the two regions. Both targets resulted in a significant reduction of dpdr symptoms, even with a single session, by about 30% *regardless* of target region. More specifically, for the VLPFC five out of the eight patients were responders (partial), defined as symptom reduction of at least 25%. For the TPJ, of nine patients, four were partial responders and one was a full responder.

After this initial finding, the group proceeded to conduct a TMS treatment study, which consisted of up to 20 treatment sessions in seven patients whose DDD was resistant to medications.[27] This study was not randomized or controlled; in methodology lingo it's called a "consecutive case series." The brain target was only the right VLPFC. After treatment, there was an average 44% reduction in dpdr symptom severity; only one patient did not respond, four were partial responders, and two were full responders. As expected, response was greater than in the earlier study that consisted of a single session. Also of interest, other types of dissociative symptoms, as measured by the Dissociative Experiences Scale, did not change. The 44% response magnitude in this study was very similar to the 49% response reported for the right TPJ in the New York study.

It's readily apparent that our TMS treatment findings for DDD so far appear quite promising: in two studies targeting two different brain regions, patients' dpdr severity approximately halved. Unfortunately, no further TMS treatment trials have been reported as of 2022 in DDD. One would like to see larger, randomized, and placebo-controlled ("sham TMS") trials. A treatment study *combining both targets* in a single protocol would be of great interest, as both yielded positive results.

Regardless, we have now added a new tool in our biological arsenal for treating DDD. TMS is not approved for DDD by the U.S. Food and Drug Administration, just as no medications are—such approvals require substantially more work and treatment data. Still, in clinical practice, DDD patients who have proven resistant to numerous medications now have the option to try TMS treatment. It is readily available across many TMS treatment centers and can adopt the same specifications and parameters that were used in the research studies. TMS has a very good safety profile, so there is little concern about pursuing a more experimental treatment. On the other hand, it does require a significant time commitment (daily sessions for a minimum of three weeks), and unfortunately can be prohibitively expensive for many.

Beyond Somatic Treatments

Can medications, however effective, do the job alone? Most experts believe not. Still, people who can trace their onset to a specific incident such as the use of drugs, or who view the condition as purely biologically based and having occurred for no apparent reason, are likely to resist such thinking. "I know what happened, and all the talk in the world isn't going to make it better," is the typical conclusion. And, for the person who once had a strong, independent self, the "stigma" of mental illness and "blind" long-term reliance on a therapist can be quite a deterrent. "I don't want to become dependent on therapy" is, regrettably, a common saying. Yet what psychotherapy actually entails is not well known to many, despite preconceptions, and has broadened and richened in our times.

Even psychiatrists who routinely prescribe medications and are well versed in psychopharmacology agree that in the case of DDD, an effective combination of medicine and psychotherapy is a wiser course of treatment. "People who have suffered with DDD for years, and have tried everything, think of the possibility of a cure with a year or two of psychotherapy are anxious to take that chance," Dr. Torch, an Atlanta-based psychiatrist and DDD expert, says. One DDD patient, who did find relief through a variety of medications, expressed his ongoing dissatisfaction: "Medications have helped my depersonalization a lot, but they've been like showing a cross to a vampire. The cross keeps him at bay, but I'm still looking for that spike in the heart that will finish him off." In the next three chapters, we'll look at some of the psychotherapy theories and techniques that, with or without medication, attempt to deal a more crippling blow to this sometimes treatment-resistant disorder.

11

What to Expect
when Starting Psychotherapy

Everything in this world has a hidden meaning.

—Nikos Kazantzakis

People with depersonalization/derealization disorder (DDD) often arrive for their first consultation confused and worried about what ails them. It is not uncommon for them to have already visited practitioners who did not diagnose their condition accurately, or possibly labeled their symptoms as a form of anxiety, depression, or stress. They may even have been told that they suffer from DDD, but the clinician confessed to knowing little about it. Understandably, such happenings can fuel confusion over one's diagnosis, or undermine confidence when embarking on a new treatment. Patients who are being seen for the first time should receive a thorough evaluation to determine whether they are indeed experiencing depersonalization/derealization (dpdr) symptoms, and whether these symptoms are part of another psychiatric condition or constitute DDD (Chapters 4 and 5).

An appropriate course of treatment can be recommended only when all applicable diagnoses are determined. In addition to a thorough chronological history of dpdr symptoms, it can be helpful to administer the Dissociative Experiences Scale and the Cambridge Depersonalization Scale at the first meeting (Chapter 3) to better appreciate the nature of the dissociative symptoms, to quantify dpdr severity, to exclude other dissociative conditions, and to hone in on the most prominent and troublesome symptom clusters (e.g., numbing, perceptual alterations, derealization etc.).

Once a clinician establishes that a particular patient is diagnosable with DDD, he/she explains to the patient why the DDD diagnosis is an appropriate

Feeling Unreal. Second Edition. Daphne Simeon and Jeffrey Abugel, Oxford University Press. © Oxford University Press 2023. DOI: 10.1093/oso/9780197622445.003.0011

one, provides basicpsychoeducational information about the nature of the disorder, especially as it relates to the particular patient, and introduces initial psychotherapeutic interventions that will help the therapy take off. The important components of DDD psychoeducation that follow can be tailored to each patient's knowledge about the condition, their particular presentation, and other psychological issues and needs.

Labeling and Normalization

Naming and appreciating dpdr symptoms for what they are can be tremendously relieving. It can also be useful to frame symptoms on the continuum on which they occur. This may range from transient and common responses to stress, and the protective function served by the sensory and emotional distancing from overwhelming experience, to the more persistent syndrome meeting the threshold for the disorder of DDD. Though the latest edition of the *Diagnostic and Statistical Manual of Mental Disorders* (*DSM-5-TR*) does not specify a minimal duration for the disorder, it makes clinical sense, as a rough guideline, to diagnose a patient with DDD if they have been experiencing dpdr independently from other conditions for at least two or three months. This is especially important if a patient is in the process of recovery from an episode of another disorder, such as major depression or panic disorder. It is not unusual for associated dpdr symptoms to remit more gradually than other hallmark symptoms of the particular disorder.

Knowing What Depersonalization Is and Isn't

It is extremely helpful for patients to understand what *it is* that they are suffering from, especially if dpdr experiences have previously been dismissed or simply misunderstood. Many people experiencing depersonalization have never encountered another person suffering from the same thing, although the internet has substantially lessened this kind of isolation. Giving the syndrome a name and describing to patients how it typically presents, what brings it on, and what can be expected in the future can be tremendously reassuring. Equally relieving is the reassurance that depersonalization, no matter how severe, never evolves into something different or even worse—people with dpdr never actually "lose their minds" (a common concern) or become psychotic or schizophrenic from it. Additionally, DDD does not involve irreversible brain damage, another common fear: it is no more or less structural than any other psychiatric disorder, where alterations in brain circuits, brain function, or even isolated brain structures are commonly present.

It also helps patients to know that the course of DDD, though sometimes chronic, can be quite unpredictable. For some, episodes can last for weeks, months, or even a few years, and then gradually fade. Often, each person's unique history is the *best* predictor of future course. Sometimes, people can get caught up in the guilt or self-blame of what it was that they initially might have done, or failed to do, that precipitated the illness—whether it was smoking marijuana, or allowing themselves to be subjected to severe prolonged stress and not doing something about it. It is very therapeutic to overcome the exaggerated sense of responsibility frequently associated with these thoughts and feelings. Ultimately, people do all kinds of things for all kinds of reasons, and these may or may not result in lasting symptoms. What happens is in one sense fortuitous, and often beyond our control or our best predictions.

Patients may even be encouraged, where appropriate, to share some of their depersonalization experiences with others. The secrecy, fear, and shame that often prevents people with DDD from communicating their suffering to others can be quite striking. Each person has their own reasons, which can be discussed. If a patient decides to open up to a trusted other, there can be a liberating sense of overcoming the barrier of a hidden illness that the person fears someone else will be unable to grasp or may misconstrue as madness. Although this may not bring about immediate improvement, it may help restore a basic sense of *connectedness* that is important to everyone's wellbeing, and especially important to people who are already feeling detached from others because of the unusual nature of their symptoms.

What Caused It?

Patients often ask this rather obvious question in their first meeting with a clinician. The answer, however, is more complex and less straightforward than the question might imply. When thinking about any psychiatric syndrome, we typically cannot isolate a *single* "cause." Rather, we think in terms of underlying vulnerabilities, both genetic and environmental, and earlier life events and adversities, coupled with more proximal precipitating life events and states of mind. This model is a helpful one to share with patients from the start. It begins to introduce some necessary complexity for patients to consider.

Sometimes, the precipitant is relatively easy to identify, such as a frightening, overwhelming, or traumatic life change, a severe bout of depression, panic or other disorder, illicit drug use, and so on. At other times the precipitating event might be more mysterious and obscure, or even not readily identifiable. A person may be presenting, for example, after they become engaged to be married, and only in time might powerful conflicts surrounding commitment emerge. Or a person may have started a job that they thought was a positive career move, only to eventually discover that they are deeply troubled by their choice. Furthermore, proximal life events are often experienced in ways that may be strongly colored, and shaped, by earlier life experiences, and those who have not previously had an opportunity to process who they are and where they came from might be particularly vulnerable. It is helpful, early on, to introduce the notion that more is likely going on than meets the eye, and that with time and treatment all the forces at play will be better understood.

Addressing the Physicality of Dpdr

The subjective physicality of dpdr symptoms has *nothing* to do with a physical or irreversible cause, yet many patients with depersonalization assume that is does. Questions like "Is my brain damaged forever?" are common. Often people extrapolate that if they feel like their mind is empty, or their head is too full, or their scalp tingles, or their vision is foggy, it all must somehow indicate brain damage or, even worse, irreversible brain damage. Proof of how powerful this conviction can be is the large number of depersonalization sufferers who have consulted numerous other medical doctors before becoming convinced, or desperate enough, to finally see a mental health professional. Ophthalmologists, neurologists, ear-nose-and-throat doctors, endocrinologists, and chronic fatigue specialists have frequently been visited in search of answers. These professionals will typically run a battery of tests pertinent to their field and expertise, which in the vast majority of cases yield no pathological findings. Finally, they will try to convince the patient that what they are experiencing is "just stress," or maybe anxiety or depression, leaving them as bewildered as they originally were, and minimally reassured.

Yet, physical manifestations of psychological states, as we well know, should not be simplistically linked to irreversible physical causes. For example, patients with clinical depression who can't eat or sleep do not have an irreversible derangement of the brain's appetite or sleep centers. Patients with panic attacks who suffer from shortness of breath do not have physical damage to the brain's respiratory centers, and so on. Psychoeducation aimed at separating the seeming physicality or persistence of dpdr symptoms from any inferences about their cause, or their reversibility, is a key early intervention in the treatment of depersonalized patients.

Who Controls Whom?

Not unlike patients with other kinds of psychological symptoms, patients with depersonalization may often feel that the symptoms (whether one, several, or alternating) are running and ruining their lives. This may be true to some extent, but typically not to the extent subjectively perceived. Therefore, it is important early on to help patients understand that they do and can have some control over their symptoms, even if limited. This is often hampered by the perception of symptoms as constant and unfluctuating, independent of any psychological determinants that have meaning, driven solely by physical environmental factors such as sleep, lighting, level of environmental stimulation, and so on.

There are different ways of helping patients, even those who perceive their symptoms as most unwavering, to start to notice that they *do* vary, and that they can begin to make some sense of these variations. One straightforward way to help patients become more aware of fluctuations is to keep a written or mental diary of their depersonalization, take note of even minimal fluctuations in intensity, and begin to relate symptom fluctuations to inner states of mind and external circumstances. Over time, patients can be helped to put more sophisticated labels on their experiences, from the simple stressed or depersonalized, to saddened, angered, overwhelmed, frightened, and so forth. Patients can also start to use various cognitive-behavioral techniques to help modulate the intensity of their symptoms (see next chapter). If these techniques meet with any initial degree of success, even transient or partial, patients come to appreciate that their symptoms do *not* entirely have a life of their own but can be modulated, albeit to varying degrees.

The Heritability Fear: Will I Pass It On?

Both men and women who suffer from depersonalization sometimes express worry about whether their children are more likely to develop the condition. Although the definitive answer may not be fully known, generally speaking, clinicians can be reassuring that from all that we do know, the likelihood of this occurring is quite low. For one, although there have been no formal family studies that interviewed the relatives of those with depersonalization, the reports of depersonalized patients, whether in clinical practice or research studies, rarely reveal parents or siblings who have experienced dpdr. There have been only three studies examining the heritability of dissociation (though not depersonalization specifically), and they had conflicting results (Chapter 7). Though it appears that there is some heritability to normative dissociation, the evidence for pathological dpdr heritability is not there. So, although no one can reassure a person with depersonalization that it will never surface in their children, it appears to be less likely than for many other psychiatric conditions, and in fact rather unlikely.

A particular worry for women may be whether their dpdr will flare up during a future pregnancy, especially if they had a prior experience where this was the case. An additional worry for women can be how they will be able to engage with their infant in a real and genuine way when they are feeling disconnected, numb, and just going through the motions. We are able, to a reasonable degree, to address both of these troubling concerns. Regarding pregnancy, we have no systematic data for DDD like we do for depression and other disorders. However, it is reasonable to think that if pregnancy was consistently associated with worsened dpdr, we would likely know it. Anecdotally, we have reports of pregnancy where dpdr symptoms either improved or worsened. During pregnancy, exacerbation or new onset of depression or anxiety always has the potential to fuel existent or new-onset dpdr, so symptoms of *all* types must be monitored carefully in a pregnancy and treated accordingly.

A new mother who has dpdr can be highly distraught by the sense of disconnection from her baby. There is some solace to be found in the fact that inner experience and relating to others are separate, especially in a relationship that is mutual but by definition asymmetrical: the mother's role is to take care of the baby, regardless and beyond her state of mind, and many mothers share this sentiment. A mother who is loving, caring, and engaged to the reasonable degree that she can be, even if her experiences feel unreal and her feelings are dampened, will likely cause no harm to her baby. The mother may find herself enjoying motherhood less, but this is a partly separate matter, though a very important one. Ongoing psychotherapy can be particularly helpful to women navigating a painful, and critical, period such as this.

Keeping a Diary

Diary keeping can help patients become more aware of fluctuations in their symptoms, as well as become more mindful of feelings, thoughts, actions, and circumstances that affect their symptoms. It can be an invaluable technique at the start, allowing a person to better monitor and make sense of their experience, thus gaining some initial sense of mastery and control. The simplest version of the diary involves keeping a daily log, on the phone or wherever else is convenient, charting dpdr intensity for the day on a 0-to-10 scale (0 being none and 10 being the worst ever for the particular person). The average, maximum, and minimum for each day is charted. For the maximum and minimum, patients can also chart the time of day, and write a brief note about their state of mind at the time and the context surrounding the moment.

The patient and therapist can review the diary together at their next session, and almost unfailingly, patterns begin to be uncovered. The external events and internal states associated with the fluctuations in depersonalization, even tiny ones, become more apparent. And this increasing awareness can be put to use. First, a patient realizes that the dpdr is not simply a flat and unvarying line (this is rarely the case). Second, a patient gains an emergent sense of mastery and hope: if dpdr can get worse, it can also get better, and if it can get better, it can get even better over time—nothing is fixed in stone. Third, meaning is introduced: things are not happening at random. Fourth, circumstances that tend to lighten the symptoms can be uncovered, understood, and fostered (to the degree that they are reasonably adaptive), whereas conditions that worsen the symptoms can be understood, avoided, or replaced with more tolerable and adaptive options.

In his first meeting with the therapist (and first time in therapy), James agreed to keep a diary, which the two began to explore together over the next two sessions. It turned out that over time, James's depersonalization would peak to an 8, or drop to a 2. James had some interesting stories to share surrounding his more intense dpdr experiences, mostly having to do with his superiors at work. The stories focused on times when he felt powerless and emasculated in the midst of potential confrontations. James got stuck and frozen whenever interests and needs had to be reconciled, his and others'. A theme began to emerge having to do with asserting himself versus placating others, and he felt more unreal when acutely gripped by this conflict. What the conflict was all about was something to better understand.

Obsessions, Compulsions, and Depersonalization: Is it Still There?

Not all patients with depersonalization obsess over their symptoms, but a good number do. For some, this can be one of the more extreme and damaging manifestations of the condition. They may spend countless hours ruminating about the nature of human existence and its illusionary qualities. They may repeatedly check their perceptions hundreds of times throughout the day to determine how real or unreal they are at any moment. They may obsess over a long list of possible causes of the condition. They may endlessly attack themselves for smoking marijuana and wondering how things might have played out if they hadn't. They may examine their hand repeatedly to determine if it looks any more or less real than the last time. They may check their vision to decide if things look more or less foggy. Some patients are utterly consumed, and will admit that they think about it nonstop, "24/7" in their own words. Incessant ruminations are a tortured state of mind.

Like other types of obsessions, those about depersonalization serve no useful purpose. They reflect the overwhelming preoccupation with, and fear of, the altered way of experiencing. But they also unwittingly channel the worry into magical thinking of sorts—trying to better understand, undo or prevent, or somehow discover the unknown solution that will take it all away. But in reality, obsessing only exacerbates *any* symptom or experience that is being obsessed about, including dpdr. It is repetitive, circular, needless, and fruitless, and at its worse dysregulating and self-traumatizing.

It's important when first meeting a person with DDD to determine if obsessions or compulsions surrounding the dpdr are present—the shapes and forms they take, their frequency and intensity, and how they may be fueling the dpdr and interfering with life in general. In understanding a patient's distress, it is helpful to separate the subjective dpdr experiences from the obsessional overlay. Sometimes patients may not spontaneously bring up the obsessing; they may not think it is relevant or they may take it as an inevitable given. When the experiences are pronounced enough, a patient may feel distracted and preoccupied even in the midst of the appointment that they long awaited. Some patients will say that the obsessional overlay is more disturbing that the dpdr itself.

Meaning Making

Nothing can be more helpful and empowering than *making sense* of something that appears to make no sense at all. This is true of most things for sentient humans, and it is no different for depersonalization. As we've already noted, sometimes the physicality of dpdr, its out-of-the-blue onset, or its unwavering course regardless of how one is otherwise feeling might give the impression that the symptoms have little to do with meaning. But this is definitely not so. The more one gets to know people with DDD, the more one is struck by the complex and deeper meanings underlying the symptoms. Accordingly, uncovering, understanding, and working through the meanings concealed within the symptoms can have great therapeutic impact for many patients.

Patients may come to the initial evaluation quite clueless about what they're experiencing. It may seem that their depersonalization just set in one day, an ordinary day no different from any other. Yet, careful exploration often reveals, even from the first meeting, that the ordinary was not so ordinary; compelling precipitants may become apparent. The detached and unreal nature of the depersonalization experience inherently disrupts the capacity to contemplate real and meaningful connections between life events and the ways these are being experienced. A depersonalized individual can feel so detached that, automatically, almost as if on purpose, symptoms break the link to relevant meanings. For these reasons, it is particularly important to introduce from the start the notion that symptoms carry hidden meaning—this, of course, is the guiding principle of psychodynamic therapy. If just one pre-liminary hypothesis about meaning can be reasonably formulated from the first encounter, even if partial and incomplete, it can be very useful to lay it out and talk about it. Doing this helps a patient become more curious and begin to reflect on their inner world, combats "randomness," introduces mentalization (the capacity to reflect on one's own mind and the minds of others), and provides a fruitful framework for future therapy work.

12

Cognitive-Behavioral and Mindfulness-Based Psychotherapy

For there is nothing either good or bad, but thinking makes it so.
—Shakespeare

Rationale for Cognitive-Behavioral Therapy in Depersonalization/Derealization Disorder

Cognitive-behavioral therapy (CBT) seeks to identify and change distorted thinking patterns and behaviors as the main means of achieving symptom change, as opposed to psychodynamic psychotherapy, which concentrates on the exploration of feelings, conflicts, past and present connections, and the unconscious aspects of the mind. Cognitive characteristics that typify chronic depersonalization have long been known, such as catastrophic fears about the illness, obsessive ruminations, and hypochondriasis.

In 2003, the U.K. group put forth a comprehensive cognitive-behavioral model for understanding depersonalization/derealization disorder (DDD). The article, published in the journal *Behaviour Research and Therapy*, proposed that since transient depersonalization is a common occurrence, a CBT approach to chronic depersonalization/derealization (dpdr) symptoms need account for the mechanisms by which the symptoms are maintained and perpetuate in some individuals, but not in others.[1] Elaine Hunter's approach was based on the premise that " . . . there is substantial support for the conceptualisation of DPD [DDD] as an anxiety disorder" (p. 1454).[1] Hence the rationale for a CBT approach to treating DDD, modeled after the anxiety disorders.

A priori, anyone whose feels unreal and detached from the self or from surroundings is experiencing dissociation. While Hunter and colleagues

Feeling Unreal. Second Edition. Daphne Simeon and Jeffrey Abugel, Oxford University Press. © Oxford University Press 2023. DOI: 10.1093/oso/9780197622445.003.0012

acknowledged that subjective detachment from the external world and from one's own mental processes places DDD patients in the realm of dissociation, they also stressed that primary characteristics of other dissociative disorders—such as amnesia and identity alteration—are absent in DDD. Also, unlike other dissociative disorders where there is a pattern of shifting between non-dissociative and dissociative states, chronic dpdr can be continuous and unremitting. Furthermore, they pointed out the high co-occurrence of disorders characterized by high anxiety, such as panic, generalized anxiety disorder, posttraumatic stress disorder, obsessive-compulsive disorder, and hypochondriasis. Finally, the U.K. group has traditionally minimized the role of trauma and other adversities in the genesis of DDD.

Following these observations, Hunter and colleagues essentially conceptualized DDD as an anxiety-type disorder, treatable through anxiety-informed CBT principles adapted for dpdr symptoms. Of course, in the final analysis, it hardly matters to a suffering patient which classification their disorder should rightfully be in, or what the rationale of a treatment might be, as long as it *works*. DDD, like the head of Medusa, is a thing unto itself that can bite you any number of ways without the slightest concern about the genus to which it belongs. But a theoretical rationale must back up any therapy formulation, and is worth understanding.

The Anxiety-Based CBT Model

Based on the above conceptualizations, the U.K. group proposed that some individuals who experience temporary dpdr may attribute it to a variety of stressful situations and pay little attention to it; the absence of preoccupation and worry leads to the smooth and timely decrease in symptoms as the situational factors resolve. Other individuals, however, may catastrophically misinterpret their transient symptoms, taking them to mean that they are going crazy, about to lose control, or become invisible, or have an irreversible brain disease. These kinds of thinking understandably lead to an increase in anxiety, which in turn fuels the continuation and worsening of depersonalization symptoms, in effect locking in the vicious cycle.

These individuals develop a range of *cognitive biases* and *avoidance behaviors* that further serve to maintain their symptoms. Situations that exacerbate the symptoms—for example, social situations or crowded overstimulating settings—start to be avoided. The sense of detachment can also lead to diminished motivation and difficulty enjoying previously pleasurable activities, resulting in low mood, frustration, and decreased engagement with life. Sufferers also adopt so-called *safety behaviors*—behaviors believed to help prevent feared outcomes. Patients try hard to act "normal" and appear engaged, only leading to an increase of their sense of unreality. They also develop *attentional biases*, such that an increase in self-monitoring and in symptom-focusing lead to a *hyperawareness* of their mental state, and to an increased likelihood of perceiving *threat* in any situation that could potentially intensify symptoms. They may develop a tendency toward *heightened introspection* and over-intellectualization of their experiences, often along existential lines, which only accentuate the emotional detachment.

Using the model just described, a first (and as of now the only) study using CBT to treat DDD was conducted at the Institute of Psychiatry.[2] The study enrolled 21 patients with DDD who were treated individually with CBT. The treatment trial was what is known as an "open" one: there was no control group of DDD patients who received a non-CBT treatment for comparison. Most of the patients (17) were taking medication for DDD, and about two-thirds were experiencing significant anxiety and/or depression. The CBT therapy consisted of about 13 sessions, centered on three main components: re-interpreting dpdr symptoms in less threatening ways; decreasing avoidant behaviors; and reducing hyperawareness and symptom monitoring. There was overall improvement by the end of treatment, at which point six patients no longer met criteria for the disorder. On average, dpdr severity in the patient group declined by a modest 20%, based on the numbers reported. Importantly, the treatment gains were maintained and even somewhat greater at a six-month follow-up.

Ultimately, clinicians may choose to take a primarily CBT approach in treating a patient with DDD, especially if they are CBT specialists. Or they may be more eclectic and incorporate CBT elements into a broader therapy that blends more than one approach. We started out with an explication of the anxiety-based CBT model for the disorder, as this is the only one currently published. However, it is important to note that a clinician need not fully espouse the anxiety-based model in formulating cognitive, behavioral, and mindfulness interventions tailored to each DDD patient.

Targeting DDD Cognitions

In this section we distinguish between anxiety-driven, negatively distorted thoughts and the process of overthinking in and of itself, which in people with

DDD often takes the form of obsessional, intrusive ruminations about their condition. Despite some overlap (those who catastrophically worry are more prone to develop obsessions and compulsions), different CBT approaches are used to target anxious catastrophizing versus obsessional ruminating.

Challenging catastrophic assumptions involves the gradual deconstruction of the various catastrophic ideas about depersonalization, through psychoeducation, evidence gathering, and the formulation of alternative and more normative assumptions. Here is a list (and not a complete one) of some common catastrophic cognitions encountered in DDD.

1. I'm going crazy.
2. I'm losing control.
3. My brain is irreversibly damaged.
4. I live in an alternate reality.
5. I no longer have a self.
6. I'm becoming invisible.
7. Nothing exists or is real.
8. This is the worst condition in the world; I'd rather have depression or cancer.
9. I know this will never go away.
10. I can't concentrate or remember anything.

Let's now take a closer look at these terrifying thoughts, examine the evidence, and reframe them into counter-cognitions that are more normalized and reality-based—we have already addressed these at different points throughout the book.

1. There is no evidence that people with DDD "go crazy," and we know that dpdr never evolves into psychosis, or dementia, or any other condition for that matter.
2. I have never so far lost control as a result of my dpdr, and therefore I am not likely to. I am overwhelmed, so it is no wonder I feel like I will lose control.
3. Science has not shown irreversible brain damage in DDD. Like in many other psychiatric conditions, I may have reversible changes in my brain chemistry and activity.
4. I live in the same reality as everyone else, and I know it, but it feels very different.

5. I do have a self, but at this moment I am having trouble owning and experiencing my self like I did before.
6. I am not invisible, but it's harder for me to see myself; others can see me just the same.
7. I exist no more or less than everybody else, and the ultimate nature of existence has nothing to do with my dpdr.
8. Comparing maladies is futile, and unless I'm suffering from something I cannot really know what it would really feel like. I did not know how dpdr feels until it happened.
9. No one can exactly predict the future of my dpdr, but I have confidence that with treatment I will get better.
10. My attention and memory feel off, but there is no evidence from cognitive studies that I have any major cognitive impairment.

To successfully implement alternative cognitions, the patient works with their clinician to determine which ones are most prevalent and troubling, and to examine their own "personal evidence" for their beliefs. Different people can have very different evidence and sources on which they base their beliefs, or hardly any evidence at all. Next, they work together to formulate an alternative, less catastrophic, and more reality-based belief, tailoring it in content and phrasing to what best makes sense for the patient. At some point any patient will invariably say "this makes sense": it is then helpful to take note of the revised cognition. In this way, every time the patient revisits a catastrophic cognition, its "saner" version is readily at hand.

If it proves helpful, patients can keep a cognitive diary, and record a daily 0-to-10 rating for how successful they were in normalizing their catastrophic cognitions. Patients may also use daily homework sheets in which they record the negative thoughts, the evidence for and against them, and the corrected thoughts. However, caution needs to be exercised in doing the "homework," since people with DDD are prone to overthinking, and to researching and revisiting all the evidence that might prove or disprove their worst fears. Maybe there is something on the internet that they missed the last time around. Maybe there is some new information on the internet today that wasn't there last week. And so forth. Though these scenarios may sound far-fetched, they are not unusual. One needs to be especially mindful, when reformulating cognitions, not to get carried away with searching for and reviewing evidence. There is nothing new to be found, and a patient hopefully trusts their therapist's knowledge. The evidence is quite simple and clear, and when sessions become consumed with reviewing and repeating evidence as if it's the first time, it's time to step back and reflect: "I've been over this many times before, and I must admit that it is pretty simple and clear. Maybe I'm having difficulty hearing it and accepting it."

Obsessional preoccupations surrounding the symptoms and the disorder may also be a factor. DDD patients may first present for treatment with elaborate obsessional thinking, sometimes accompanied by ritualistic behaviors, such as checking over and over to determine whether the symptoms have changed (e.g., if one looks any more or less real in the mirror, or one feels less or more numbed out than the last time they checked a few minutes or a half an hour ago). At times, the extent of the preoccupations can be 24/7, occupying massive mental space, causing psychic torment, and greatly distracting from a person's ability to attend to all else in their life. In these situations, it is not unusual for a patient to admit that their preoccupation with the symptoms is in fact *worse* than the symptoms themselves. For example, if asked to do the usual 0-to-10 rating, a patient might say that symptoms are at a 4 but ruminations are at an 8. In this case, it is useful to include separate ratings for subjective experience and ruminations in the daily diary, as a reminder of this important distinction.

A variety of CBT techniques akin to those used for the treatment of obsessive-compulsive disorder are useful in tackling dpdr-focused obsessions and compulsions. *Thought management, exposure and response prevention*, and *distraction* are some of the standard techniques. Patients can learn to "catch" themselves as soon as they become aware that they are once again obsessing. They cannot simply "block" the thinking, or they would have already done so, but they can mindfully attend to their thoughts from a fresh perspective: "Here I go obsessing again, but there is nothing new. I am wasting time and energy and causing myself a lot of distress." Or, "I will take mental note of my thought, and accept it as the non-event that it really is; its content is not worth contemplating yet again." Or, "I am not ignoring my thoughts but putting them in their rightful place." The phrases can be tailored to each patient's preference and can be recorded, so they are readily available whenever they're needed.

In conjunction with this process, it can be helpful for a patient to then engage in a distracting task. What the task will be is a matter of individual preference, as well as what is appropriately doable in different settings. It can range from engaging in a simple task at hand that the patient needs or wants to do but has been postponing or avoiding, to simple but absorbing tasks like playing a game on one's phone, counting up by 3s to 100, or counting objects of a certain color indoors or outdoors.

Exposure and response prevention is a central technique to treating repetitive thinking and behaviors. Exposure involves confronting all the cues that trigger dpdr-related obsessions and compulsions. It is done gradually, starting with triggers that provoke lower distress and moving on to more challenging ones. This can be done either in one's imagination (imaginal exposure) or in real life (in vivo). Exposing oneself to one's own obsessional thoughts can be simply imaginal. A person systematically evokes the scary obsessional thought and tolerates the associated feelings until the anxiety diminishes.

Another kind of exposure is less gradual and more "flooding." One common technique is known as "loop recording." The patient uses a voice recorder (most commonly their phone these days) to record a narrative that captures their usual obsessional thinking, then plays it on a loop over and over for about 30 minutes a day. In listening, one attempts to experience the full distress of the ruminations. Over time, through what is known as systematic desensitization and habituation, the distress caused by the obsessional thinking diminishes.

When it comes to ritualistic behaviors, the approach is similar. A person with DDD learns to refrain from their usual "compulsive" behavioral response to a dpdr-related obsessional thought. For example, a patient who repeatedly looks in the mirror to check how real their face appears to them, many times throughout the day, will now resist and not look in the mirror at all, or will look the few times when it is absolutely necessary (e.g., putting on make-up) and for only as long as it takes to simply do the task at hand. In this way, the obsessional thinking about the realness of one's face will diminish over time, as the ritualistic response that has been maintaining and reinforcing it is prevented.

It takes effort not to engage with obsessions and compulsions, and patients can rate in their daily diary how successful they were in resisting, as well as how successful they were in controlling their thinking and behaviors. A pattern will emerge with time, and when the techniques are used consistently the ratings will go down.

Targeting DDD Avoidant Behaviors

When dpdr symptoms set in and more so over time, some DDD patients develop a range of avoidance behaviors as a way of dealing with all the situations that trigger their symptoms. For example, a person may start avoiding stressful social encounters, job meetings, physical settings such as crowded places, unknown places, overstimulating places, bright sunlight days, twilight hours, fluorescent lighting, and so on. At its most extreme, a minority of patients become severely agoraphobic and homebound. All these behaviors are invariably maladaptive, as they impede a person's regular routines, socialization, connectedness to others, work performance, and the like. And, most importantly, avoidance is self-perpetuating and self-augmenting by nature: the immediate relief that it brings, whether real or imagined (since the situation was avoided one cannot be certain each time), only leads to more avoidance. Some patients are very pained by all they are avoiding and missing out on; others may have lost sight of how constricted their lives have become.

The standard technique for reducing avoidance is known as *graded exposure*. The therapist and patient together formulate a hierarchy of counter-avoidant behaviors, rated from 1 (easiest) to 10 (hardest) in terms of difficulty. The patient then begins to practice the counter-avoidant behavior rated as 1 (e.g., walking around the block twice a day for someone who is otherwise homebound). For any exposure to succeed and lead to habituation, so that the behavior becomes easier and easier, it must be regularly practiced. After a new behavior is mastered and the dpdr it evokes decreases to a tolerable level, the client is ready to move to the next level of difficulty. Though exposure can be quite frightening, a person invariably experiences satisfaction in remastering ordinary daily behaviors that have been relinquished in fear of the disorder, and this in and of itself has an empowering impact.

Targeting DDD Hyperawareness and Self-Monitoring

Another common feature of the disorder is many DDD sufferers' tendency to become increasingly hyperaware and selectively focused on their symptoms and their altered self-experience. This attentional honing-in inevitably results in a marked magnification of perceptions, and creates cognitive biases. The slightest worsening of blurriness and fog, or spaciness, or empty-mindedness does not escape notice, whereas conversely any lightening up of the symptoms goes unnoticed. It can be helpful to normalize what hyperawareness is about, because it happens all the time and in all kinds of contexts. For example, many people have floaters, and the more they focus on them the more floaters they see. Or many people have pain and aches, and the more they focus on the physical discomfort, the stronger it feels. The simple explanation for this is that our perceptions are not simply peripheral (registered by the relevant organs), but there are complex brain mechanisms at work that amplify or dampen our perceptions at any given moment in time.

Hyperawareness can be helped by a variety of *refocusing, grounding,* and *mindfulness* techniques. Despite their different names all these techniques overlap in that they manipulate and alter attentional processes, thus breaking the cycle of dpdr-sensation–focused attention. Refocusing techniques involve willful retraining and control of attention, for example promoting divided over selective attention with a distraction task. In this regard, DDD patients might feel encouraged by a reminder that, as a group, they are quite skilled in dividing attention (Chapter 7). This technique is similar to that commonly used to manage chronic pain. The distraction can take the form of attending to other bodily or environmental sensory inputs that are unrelated to DDD, such as one's breathing or muscle tone, or the texture and coloring of an out-side object regardless of its blurriness. The competing sensory stimuli require attentional dividing, and lessen the narrow focus through the lens of dpdr.

Grounding generally refers to feeling more present, connected, and able to process information. Grounding techniques abound and can be readily searched by anyone. Many of us ground ourselves throughout the day without even realizing it, by slowing down, sighing, take a few deep breaths, or mo-mentarily emptying our minds and taking in a beautiful sunset. Grounding techniques vary according to the modality employed (sensory, physical, emotional) or the condition targeted (panic, PTSD, dissociation, etc.), and ultimately need to be shaped to fit each person's preferences, facilities, and responsiveness.

One common form of *sensory grounding* is the 5-4-3-2-1 method. A person searches for, acknowledges, and engages with five things they can see, four things they can touch, three things they can hear, two things they can smell, and one thing they can taste. These can be objects in the immediate envi-ronment or parts of one's body. *Physical grounding* is body-focused and can involve various practices, deep breathing being a central one. A common exercise involves relaxing the body in a restful position, closing the eyes, placing one hand on the chest and the other on the belly, inhaling slowly and deeply into the belly to the count of 4, holding in and feeling the breath to the count of 7, and slowly exhaling all the air to the count of 8. An im-agery component can be added, such as a restful and safe place, or a thought or feeling that one can breathe in, hold, and then let go. Other physical grounding techniques include feeling the weight of one's feet on the ground, or the pressure of one's body against a chair or a mat. *Emotional grounding* involves reminding oneself that one is safe in the moment, though it may not feel like it, or that the past belongs to the past and not the present; visualizing a safe place through imagery; or clenching one's fist to grab on to a distressing feeling, squelching it, and then releasing it and letting it fly away.

All the above techniques aimed at reducing dpdr hyperawareness need, as always, to be tailored to the individual. One element of this tailoring, when it comes to DDD, is to consider adding or emphasizing an *emotional component* to any exercise, given the difficulties with feeling and emotional processing. As we've described throughout, hypoemotionality and numbing are key features of the disorder. Adding feelings to anything we are engaged in helps bring it, and us, more to life. For example, when willfully shifting attention to alternative perceptions and sensations, it can help to imbue them with emotional vividness, texture, and color, as much as possible. Simply acknowledging the 5-4-3-2-1 objects is not the same as truly experiencing them, taking them in, and magnifying the momentary emotional experience associated with them (e.g., the exuberance of smelling a peach, or the comfort of smelling one's favorite pillow). Even looking in the mirror and intently identifying with the realness of the reflected self can sometimes help, in conjunction with a self-affirmation like "this is Me!"

For those patients who are most troubled by visual dpdr, use of nonvisual modalities may help with grounding. Closing the eyes and intently listening to an emotionally intense and loved piece of music, smelling a favorite aroma, or tasting a special treat may work better for some than the visual. Willful immersion in the senses can be grounding for many. For those who feel numbed to touch, willfully touching and engaging with different parts of the body can be helpful, like squeezing an earlobe, pressing down on the palm of the hand, or massaging the forearms—every patient can discover their own physical manipulation that can help ground them. Physical sensation bordering on pain, within reason, can on occasion be helpful as well (e.g., snapping a rubber band on the wrist). One patient who had been depersonalized for many years described in his initial evaluation that he had felt "real" just twice during his long illness, once when he experienced intense romantic love, and once when he was accidentally slammed by the shutting subway car doors and felt intense pain.

Mindfulness-Based Therapy

In their book *Overcoming Depersonalization Disorder*, Drs. Donnelly and Neziroglu outlined an adaptation of Acceptance and Commitment Therapy

(ACT) for DDD.[3] The main premise of ACT is an acceptance of suffering in the present moment, all the while committing to pursuing what is most important in one's life. Wise and commonsensical, it can also be met with disappointment, resentment, and resistance by sufferers if understood simplistically as some version of giving up. ACT's message is much subtler and deeper and in fact is the opposite of giving up. Human suffering is an inevitable and inherent part of the human condition, whatever shape or form it takes at any particular time, and fighting the suffering or postponing life until it's over is counterproductive and demoralizing, and fuels further suffering.

ACT is a mindfulness-based therapy. Acceptance means owning the bad and the difficult along with the good and the pleasant, and recognizing that life is always a mixed bag, sometimes more so than others. Pathologizing suffering and negatively labeling it as inherently "bad" makes it even harder to tolerate and work with. The model promotes psychological flexibility, the willingness to acknowledge and equally embrace all types of feelings and experiences, including the more disturbing and uncomfortable ones. In contrast, psychological inflexibility constricts a person and their options, making it harder to move forward in life irrespective of the suffering that one is experiencing at any given time.

ACT centers around six organizing principles that can be readily applied to DDD.[3]

Cognitive Fusion

This process refers to accepting what the mind is experiencing as the *only* reality: "if I think and feel it, it must be true." For example, if a depressed person feels utterly hopeless, then indeed there is zero hope; this is not so, of course. Similarly, if a person with DDD feels or believes they are losing their mind, this is in fact not so. However, ACT does not emphasize information gathering and lists of supporting and negating evidence, like CBT. Rather, it proposes that one embrace the fundamental fact that the human mind is complex, ever-changing, and fallible, and recognize that fragility and vulnerability need to be understood and respected, but not bought into. Accepting one's state of mind and at the same time maintaining a healthy observing distance from the mind's contents in any given moment is the essence of mindfulness. In other words, DDD sufferers who feel they are going crazy must both recognize the painful subjective experience and realize that their mind is not the only truth, and that alternative perspectives exist and are just as real as what the power of the mind dictates.

Identifying the Self with the Illness

Notice that a person who is suffering from cancer will say, "I have cancer," yet the person who has depression or DDD will say, "I am depressed" or "I am depersonalized." The identification of one's whole being with the mental affliction has already occurred, even if it is not an intentional or conscious one. The DDD sufferer could just as easily say, "I have DDD." The distinction may sound superficial or trivial, but it's fundamental. Any human being is more than the sum of their afflictions, and to experience it otherwise is a step toward objectification, a problem already inherent to DDD. The ramification and psychic cost of equating the self with the condition is that other aspects of the self are dimmed and become less accessible and important. One's desires, goals, and actions are more and more driven by the DDD self-definition. Such a path is clearly maladaptive, and ACT takes the approach of helping people remember and reconstruct who they are, despite their illness.

Rumination and Worry

Worrying and obsessing, which we already covered in the CBT section, not only result in self-torment but also take the person out of the present moment. The focus on what is wrong and when it will get better is wasted, fruitless mental energy that is all-consuming and detracts from engaging in just about anything else. If a person looks back on how things have played out so far, they realize that ruminating never brings relief or new insight—rather than being constructive, as it may feel in the moment, it is destructive.

Experiential Avoidance

As already discussed in the CBT section, DDD sufferers will go to great length to avoid or escape their distressing internal dpdr experiences. To break this avoidance cycle, there needs to be willingness to tolerate frustration and discomfort. Otherwise, no matter how thoughtfully a hierarchical graded exposure plan is put together, it will not be executed. ACT helps to culti-vate this willingness, rather than simply focusing on the behavioral goals. It argues that increased willingness to engage in meaningful and enriching activities, even if accompanied by heightened symptoms and distress, is often a net positive proposition. Many patients will admit that though the antici-pation of engaging rather than avoiding can be very anxiety-provoking, after the fact the benefits are easier to appreciate and need to be held in mind for the next time.

Clarifying Values

The more a person can formulate and pursue their values, whatever they might be, the better equipped they will be to tolerate pain and suffering and to derive some meaning and pleasure from their lives. ACT helps patients hone in on their core values and regain a sense of their importance, so that life will be experienced as more purposeful and meaningful despite the suffering.

Narrow Behavioral Repertoire

The antidote to the ever-narrowing behavioral repertoire that can occur, to greater or lesser degrees, in those with DDD is what ACT calls "committed action." This constitutes willful action intent on pursuing all that is funda-mentally valuable to a person, ultimately bringing gratification instead of postponing living.

In summary, ACT fosters psychological growth through more neutralized and mindful self-observation; separation of one's identity from the illness; willingness to accept and endure suffering while it lasts; and formulation of values coupled with committed actions. Though ACT tackles domains sim-ilar to those in CBT, it is more focused on the person than the symptoms, providing a framework that can counteract the obstacles stemming from the symptoms. ACT could be said to be less mechanistic and more holistic than CBT, yet despite differences in philosophical tenets the two can be success-fully combined to broaden treatment options and provide greater psycholog-ical flexibility. ACT seeks to recast symptoms and allow room for an accepting and committed way of living alongside them, and despite them. Solace, gratification, and progress can be gained with this approach. It is therapeutic because it challenges the omnipotence and omniscience of symptoms—they are no longer the "be-all and end-all." Magical thinking sometimes sets in: "If I learn to live better with this, it is less likely to get better." It is hopefully obvious that such thinking is irrational.

13

Psychodynamic Psychotherapy

Psychotherapy is not making clever and apt interpretations; by and at large it is a long-term giving the patient back what the patient brings. The patient will find his or her own self, and will be able to exist and feel real.

—D. W. Winnicott

Ben

From his first visit to a therapist, 22-year-old Ben could appreciate a direct connection between the onset of his depersonalization and a precipitating event. When he was 15 his mother, whom he loved dearly, had unexpectedly died at age 58 from a heart attack. He'd had no opportunity to say goodbye. A couple of months after, depersonalization set in and persisted—though Ben did not deny the timing, he could not meaningfully relate the two happenings. Anyone deeply hurt, even devastated, he thought, should still be able to eventually recover. What was it then that led Ben to become chronically depersonalized after his loss, whereas others may not have remained symptomatic?

It turned out that Ben's mother had been a caring parent but was depressive and unfulfilled in in her personal life, something painfully evident to her son as far back as he could remember. She had lost her own parents at a young age and was married to an uninvolved and self-absorbed man who had little to offer her emotionally. Ultimately, outside of his awareness, Ben felt responsible for his mother's happiness. Only he could "bring her to life," so inevitably he failed her when she died. His inner, psychic, reality was too overwhelming to bear and left Ben feeling unreal for a long time.

Ben's therapy focused on helping him with the complexity of his feelings over his mother's loss. Beyond the grief he already knew, he uncovered that

Feeling Unreal. Second Edition. Daphne Simeon and Jeffrey Abugel, Oxford University Press. © Oxford University Press 2023. DOI: 10.1093/oso/9780197622445.003.0013

he felt very guilty, as if he had abandoned her. At first a foreign notion, with time he came to understand and embrace it. The more he talked about his life growing up, he *realized* that he harbored a lot of hurt, disappointment, and resentment for having been put, from the start, in the untenable position of feeling responsible for her wellbeing. By the third year in treatment Ben came to emotionally own that, despite his love for his mother, *in reality* a child cannot be responsible for a parent's wellbeing and he'd been dealt a pretty unfair card. In the process of discovering this new reality, his unreality symptoms steadily diminished.

Aisha

Aisha was 28, and she grew up in a home where her two parents screamed and yelled at each other much of the time. Since she was little, Aisha wondered why they stayed together. The parents' constant arguing scared her and distracted her, and as she got older she experienced it as very disrespectful to her need for peace, privacy, and safety in her own home. Despite her pleas, her parents did not appear interested in or capable of controlling their behavior when she was around. Aisha vividly recalled the first time she purposefully tried to tune them out. At around 14, she became deeply absorbed, almost hypnotized, by a concert poster on her bedroom wall, while saying in her head over and over "shut up and go away." This was her first moment of fleeting depersonalization.

After that incident and through the years, Aisha became increasingly depersonalized; her episodes became longer and more frequent. She often found it very hard to focus on tasks, and she described how she would become distracted by conversations in the background that she was not interested in yet could not block out. She had, however, found ways to tolerate her depersonalization/derealization (dpdr) without major difficulty, until the birth of her first child. Aisha soon discovered that the baby's crying triggered a similar response of depersonalizing and wanting to shut out the "noise," much to her distress and guilt. The baby had tipped the scale—though she experienced the intensity of his crying as unbearable, she did not want to filter it out. Her depersonalization grew denser, and she sought help.

A realization eventually came about in therapy. Aisha had become an expert at dividing her attention between tasks that she needed to attend to and all the noise around her that she wanted to filter out yet vigilantly felt compelled to monitor. Intrusive threats to her wellbeing were everywhere, and not surprisingly she at first experienced her therapist's interpretations as a major intrusion, to the point of almost quitting treatment. But Aisha was not a person who easily gave up, and she found ways to tolerate her therapist's efforts to help her, rather than leave the treatment and unwittingly repeat her life story. Her love for her baby was a powerful motivator.

With time, Aisha's impulse to tune out and escape diminished. She became increasingly adept at identifying the fear of being intruded on in real time, whenever it occurred, and at reflecting on its meanings. She came to recognize that sometimes when her personhood felt invaded, she needed to process her experience and make sense of it. Sometimes it was not really an intrusion in the present but an intrusion from the past—she cared about her baby and wanted to care for him. On the other hand, her boss's incessant complaining about her home life with her husband was of no interest to Aisha, and she felt increasingly entitled to set limits—it was not her problem, she realized, nor was her parents' bickering. With increasing clarity about her needs and wants came a diminution of her depersonalization symptoms.

Noah

Noah had felt depersonalized for about a year, after an extended period of severe and escalating stress. Over the past several years he had finished graduate school, worked increasingly demanding jobs, relocated three times, married, cared for his ailing parents, and was preparing to have a family of his own. Yet he was barely able to acknowledge all the pressures and expectations that he put on himself, focused solely on his drive to achieve and "move forward" in life.

Initially he described his childhood as a "normal" one, but gradually opened up to his therapist about the family dynamics. His mother was a successful self-made businesswoman who looked down on his stay-at-home writer father. She had always wanted a daughter and had told Noah so when he was little, but she had been unable to have a second child. When she felt frustrated with her husband, she became emotionally abusive to her son. She warned Noah that he and his father were alike and that he needed to watch out or he would amount to nothing, like his dad. From a young age she inflicted on her son her unchallengeable belief that people are born a certain way and not much can be done about it. When he was accepted to a good college, she chose not to financially contribute despite her means. She made it clear that her investment would likely go to waste because it would give Noah the wrong impression that life comes easy.

So, for Noah, becoming established and successful was not a mere ambition; it was a life-and-death matter of self-definition and self-worth, the path to proving his mother wrong and rising above her doubts and devaluation. All the while he was not processing his life experiences—his identity centered on pushing forward with brute force and being unstoppable. He eventually succumbed to the internal pressures and depersonalized.

Noah's treatment first concentrated on the present. It was evident to his therapist that his unreality was intimately related to the sense that he was an imposter, faking his many accomplishments yet not truly experiencing them as a part of who he was. Treatment was rocky for a while as Noah was a man of actions, not feelings. He expressed to his therapist that psycho-babble felt like a waste of time, the oral equivalent to his father's writings. Noah was deeply and negatively identified with the paternal incompetence he had been spoon-fed by his mother his whole life. Though he strove to be like his mother, he had not internalized her in a positive way: he did not want to be like her, he *had* to be like her—she was the real deal. He, at heart, was an imposter just like his father.

All this was uncovered and discussed in the therapy, though for quite a while the therapist would not have been surprised if Noah left one day and did not come back. But the therapist grew on Noah, giving him space to experience that different people have different aptitudes and pursuits, and the right to inhabit them. With the help of his therapist, Noah began to inhabit his own accomplishments, not as accidents but as genuine expressions of his interests and capabilities. All the while, Noah got more in touch with a growing resentment toward his once-idealized mother, both for her contempt for his father and for the pressures and belittlement that she had inflicted on him. Rather than performing in a compulsory fashion and feeling like a fake in the process, Noah began to feel proud of his undertakings, and to enjoy them as really his. Amid these gradual but steady changes, his depersonalization faded away.

These three nutshell treatment cases are, in one sense, just that. Every person is unique and different, and no two depersonalization/derealization disorder (DDD) psychotherapy treatments will look, or be, the same. Psychodynamic psychotherapy is tailored to the person manifesting the symptoms or disorder, not to the disorder in a vacuum. What Ben, Aisha, and Noah all had in common was the necessity to get to know, process, and change their inner workings—their present depersonalized state of mind was telling them so. Psychodynamic theory is based on the fundamental premise that outward manifestations, be they symptoms, disorders, or ways of experiencing the self and world, inevitably reflect inner problems and struggles, often unknown or only partly known to the suffering person who has not yet contended with them.

Psychodynamic psychotherapy is commonly referred to in lay terms as "open-ended therapy," "exploratory therapy," "long-term therapy," or simply "talk therapy." It involves the therapist and the patient working together to arrive at a mutual understanding of the origins of the depersonalization, the psychic forces that led to its inevitable breakthrough, its functions and meanings, and what needs to change within the self for the depersonalization to subside and for experiencing to be, and feel, more real.

On occasion patients ask, sometimes on day one, "Will I have to keep talking about my past?" Inevitably, they will, but not all the time—not because it is some expectation or rule, but because the self exists in continuity over time, ever-changing on one hand, yet rooted in its history from the very start. During the psychotherapy process, inner struggles originating in the past but still very much alive and at play in the present are identified, understood, and worked through, leading to a lessening of symptoms and promoting more adaptive ways of being, relating, and living.

Classic Psychoanalytic Reflections on Depersonalization Treatment

In the field of psychoanalysis, there exists a long, lingering, and self-perpetuating narrative surrounding some of the challenges and difficulties in treating people with primary depersonalization. The condition has not been written about extensively—a cursory search of the voluminous psychoanalytic database PEP, from the start of psychoanalysis to today, yields a mere 35 journal articles with the word "depersonalization" in their title. And even on the occasions that depersonalization was written about, perspectives were quite disparate and hard to bring together. One example is that while some theorists approached depersonalization as a psychosis or near-psychosis (which it is not), others conceptualized it as a neurosis akin to depression or phobic anxiety, and others yet as a "borderline" phenomenon—very large gaps in thinking, not to mention that psychoanalytically oriented psychotherapy does not work for psychosis and requires parameters and modifications for severe personality pathology.

However, the older theorists, who most insightfully understood depersonalization and who put much thought into how to best treat it, expressed greater optimism about psychotherapy. For example, in 1938 Bergler and Eidelberg wrote: "We think that this absolute pessimism is not justified; however, it is a prerequisite for the therapy that one knows the mechanisms and starts on the right point. Furthermore, very long time is necessary. While the analysis of a more severe case of obsession neurosis takes at least two to two and a half years, the double space of time is a requirement for the treatment of depersonalization."[1] These observations are pretty much on target, despite being articulated nearly a century ago. The therapist must have some familiarity with what DDD is about psychically; every treatment needs a point of entry. Bergler and Eidelberg were also correct in that it can take a pretty long time to break through the barriers of detachment and disengagement— sometimes it happens faster than others.

Today's patient might ask from the start, "How long do you think this therapy will take?" An exact answer would likely be inaccurate; it could also be misleading. But it is fair to tell a person with DDD, not unlike other patients in long-term therapy, that they are in for the longer haul. It could be two years at the very least, or four, or six, but the question becomes less relevant and pressing with time. Most people who experience positive changes in themselves with therapy, even when these changes are not as rapid or dramatic as they might have imagined or hoped, want to continue. Nowadays, once-weekly psychotherapy is considered standard. However, undoubtedly patients can sometimes benefit from meeting more frequently, and the therapist might recommend this in a particular phase of the treatment.

Schilder himself[2] expressed optimism about treating the condition, whether by individual or group psychotherapy. He emphasized the essence of the depersonalized condition as "a state of the personality in which the individual feels changed in comparison to his former state." He saw two components to this change, first the altered awareness of the self and the world around, and second that depersonalized individuals are no longer able to acknowledge themselves as *personalities*. One present-day patient aptly captured this drastic change as her "old self" and her "new self," succinctly expressing how unrelated the two felt. Yet she was, of course, still the same person, a notion her therapist introduced from the start. Though the split, the loss of personhood, felt, and was, subjectively real, it had its purposes and meanings. What was less evident to this patient, and to many other DDD sufferers, is that the *person* whose selfhood now feels gone was in deep trouble to begin with. It is none other than that idealized "old self" that generated the unwanted and depersonalized "new self," with the inner world even less accessible than before, masked by the dense distraction and angst of the depersonalized state of mind.

The Cattells[3] felt that traditional psychoanalysis, involving the use of the couch and no eye contact between patient and therapist, was not indicated in depersonalization because it enhanced the experience of disconnection and unreality. This is often, but not always, so. In early stages of treatment, when the therapist is struggling to break through to the patient and establish an emotional connection, the couch is usually not helpful because it facilitates the patient's exit and disengagement. Additionally, having a patient in full view makes it easier for a therapist to use all the nonverbal cues (body posture, facial expressions, gaze) to better track the patient's fluctuating levels of dpdr in a session and explore their meaning as they happen.

With time, a therapist who works with DDD gets better and better at detecting the subtle signs and nuances of a patient's degree of presence or depersonalized absence, moment to moment, in the session. As much as many patients with DDD feel that their suffering is a particularly silent one because no one sees it, it is often visible to the trained eye. Patients become more aware and curious about the waxing and waning of their depersonalization during sessions, especially when encouraged from the start in this regard. They more readily share these fluctuations with the therapist, and strive to make sense of them. In later states of treatment, when a patient is less densely depersonalized but has difficulty opening up more (e.g., talking about sexuality or shame), the couch may prove helpful.

Writing for the *British Journal of Guidance and Counselling* in the mid-1980s, Fewtrell[4] noted the powerful relief that patients experience when they are encouraged to verbalize their subjective sensations of depersonalization to their doctors or therapists, often for the very first time. It's the same relief clinicians who understand and treat DDD encounter over and over today. Levy and Wachtel[5] suggested that it can be useful for patients to temporarily learn to accept and tolerate their depersonalization, and to reframe it as a new reality rather than an unreality—a new reality reflecting inner struggles that can no longer be dismissed: "If the patient can tolerate the experience of unrealness for a time, he can make for himself a new reality which is more solidly grounded for his own needs and perceptions, and in a sense more 'real' than his old compromises were, however comfortable and familiar they might have felt" (p. 298).[5]

Depathologizing dpdr symptoms, often experienced as "the worst thing that could have happened to me," and adopting a more tolerant and *curious* stance toward them is an important early part of treatment. Depersonalization is not the enemy, though it certainly can feel like it. Rather, depersonalization is a very distressing state of mind, yet it is signaling that things have gone astray, seemingly but not truly to a point of no return.

In 1977, Frances, Sacks, and Aronoff published a paper entitled "Depersonalization: A elf-relations perspective" in the *International Journal of Psychoanalysis*.[6] At the time, the paper made an important contribution by providing a broader, more inclusive way of psychoanalytically thinking about the processes driving dpdr, conceptualized as a major disruption in self-constancy likely related to a patient's *level of personality organization*. Earlier psychodynamic writings tended to pigeonhole the personality organization associated with DDD, based on theoretical inclinations or isolated patient cases—but, in fact, one size does not fit all. We now know that DDD patients may be organized neurotically, narcissistically, or at the borderline level—personality disorder comorbidity (see Chapter 6) and clinical experience indicate that severe personality pathology is *not* predominant, but it is encountered.

The article proposed that a person depersonalizes when the "average, expectable" experience of the known "me" breaks down. And the kinds of threats to self-constancy that different people are most vulnerable to differ by level of personality organization. The article also proposed that depersonalization can strike some components of the self-structure more than others, e.g., the body-self, the thinking-self, the feeling-self, or the agent-self. Exploring meanings specific to these domains can, in fact, offer insights and inroads. One patient who had a parent with loose and ambiguous sexual boundaries predictably depersonalized surrounding her sexuality. Another patient who never came to comfortably inhabit her body felt that it just wasn't there whenever her depersonalization spiked. Yet another, who had trouble with making up his mind, was prone to "blanking" and losing his thoughts. Two treatment vignettes of patients with different levels of personality organization follow.

David

David was a 35-year-old man with schizoid personality. He had experienced a striking absence of physical and emotional warmth throughout his childhood, to the point where the self was essentially objectified, a thing rather than a person. David felt profoundly threatened by the slightest attempts of others to get close to him; any social contact exacerbated his depersonalization. When he tried to relate to others he felt as if he were losing himself, as if the invisible envelope surrounding him was starting to melt. He had trouble knowing if the thoughts and feelings he experienced in his interactions with others came from him, or from them. Metaphorically put, the "membrane" separating the self from others was highly permeable.

The first phase of David's treatment focused on helping him appreciate how his depersonalization heightened whenever his sense of separateness from others was threatened, and fusion-like experiences set in. He came to appreciate that any interaction with others, no matter how trivial, posed a grave threat to his rudimentary personhood. If he felt criticized or disliked, most often a projection on his part, his feelings of shame and danger heightened, and he depersonalized. Paradoxically, he also depersonalized when he had interactions with others that he perceived as more positive. To be wanted or liked punctured his cocoon and forced him to consider his personhood. Defensively, being a non-person, a well-oiled machine that navigated life like an automaton, was a safe, though terribly painful, adaptation to his early life. David only felt alive in his surprisingly elaborate and vivid fantasy life. Confronting the ups-and-downs of real human relationships was inconceivable, and his therapist was no exception.

For a long time, David insisted that in fact he had no relationship with his therapist; he was simply paying for intellectual formulations that would somehow magically transform him into a real person, bypassing any emotional engagement. It took a very long time for David to entertain, and begin to believe, that his therapist might actually like him, care about him, and enjoy getting to know him. The unbearable shame surrounding his unlovability began to give way, and he started to have, for the first time ever, experiences of being seen, recognized, and known for the person he was inside the machine. As frightening as these experiences were, they were also pleasurable, and the dense objectification of his personhood began to loosen up.

Haru

Haru was a middle-aged man with strong traditional values, who believed in family and making his marriage work. He had two young children, and after several years of intense doubt and angst over his deteriorating relationship with his self-absorbed and needy wife, he had made the very difficult decision to leave her. Depersonalization set in during this time and had lasted for about a year before he sought help. It was triggered by "neurotic" dynamics having to do with his feelings of guilt over betraying his wife, which reactivated a nascent conflict over Haru's earlier life with a helpless, fragile mother. Haru's therapy grappled with his feelings of betrayal and guilt toward women whom he perceived as weak and dependent on him, and whom he felt he needed to take care of but also longed to break away from. Early in treatment, he became intensely depersonalized when he dared to express his dissociated anger and contempt more freely.

Guilt and self-blame were much more comfortable for Haru, but it was his disowned rage, and the fear of it, that were depersonalizing him. He shared memories of how his mother would crumble in hurt and weep when he expressed any resentment toward her. He poignantly recalled one time when he was about nine and bravely told his mother to get her act together—he had a photographic memory of the angst in her face as she said, "I thought you loved me." His therapist helped him to realize that a child has the right to expect that parents will be able to bear and metabolize what the child is expressing. With time, Haru was able to mourn the person his mother had not been for him. His guilt and sense of betrayal lessened, and he was able to express expectations and set limits on others without depersonalizing.

The Thematic Thread of the Unreal: Self-Experiencing

How does a person come to have, in the best-case scenario, a more-or-less stable, predictable, and cohesive sense of self, a self that feels real, genuine, authentic, and inhabited? Early child development is a field of study unto itself, theoretically tackled by psychoanalysis from Freud on, and over time enriched and modified by volumes of empirical data from developmental psychologists, infant researchers, mind theorists, and the like. Models and theories aside, it's a well-established and indisputable fact that critical stages in the development of the self unfold within the first two or three years of life, laying the earliest foundations for a healthy self.

This self is boundaried and separate from others and is experienced with reasonable constancy across time and place. It is capable of knowing, containing, processing, and regulating emotions, and mentalizes (perceives and processes the ever-changing states of mind in oneself and in others).[7,8] Terms like "real"[9] "true,"[10] and "cohesive"[11] (theoretical differences aside) have attempted to capture the elusive but important notion of a *healthy core self* that has navigated early development with relative success—inevitably bound to a "facilitating environment" of "good-enough" parenting that was attuned, fostered secure attachment and felt security, and promoted mutual recognition.[12-14] Through these complex processes, thumbnail-sketched at best here, comes about the creation of that which is ultimately experienced as "Me."

Yet, people with DDD often operate in a "pretend" fashion, reminiscent of Peter Fonagy's pretend mode of mentalization.[7] It is "as if" the self, and the world in which it's embedded, are known, felt, understood, and experienced, though this is far from the case—dissociation is a state of mind of knowing and not knowing. Patients may be pretending (not consciously or intentionally) happy childhoods, caring parents, good partners, work they enjoy, known values and ambitions—if it weren't for the dpdr that took it all away.

Still, childhood may have been troubled and a parent may not have been emotionally present; one's studies or profession may be misaligned with one's interests and passions; an intimate relationship may be founded on falsehoods; there may even have been confusion surrounding one's identity—all before the symptoms set in. Inner troubles and struggles are part of human nature, and as such they are the bread and butter of psychotherapy. What is more specific to DDD is the uncertainty, doubt, confusion, and inauthenticity ("what is real?") experienced when one's inner world, and its ongoing collisions with external reality, are too frightening to ponder. There is an absence of emotional conviction surrounding personal narratives: "I don't know" is all too common, and suggests that it is too scary to genuinely experience. A self who cannot bear to reflect, examine, and know is, inevitably, a self who cannot fully experience "Me."

Along these lines, a DDD sufferer in therapy comes to know that their dpdr has meanings. It is protective and at the same time is signaling a breaking point. If one continues to disown all that is too threatening and frightening to know, the alternative (depersonalization) may grow and fester to the point of becoming unbearable as well. If phenomenologically (on the surface) a near-death accident and a more ordinary happening can elicit a similar felt experience, there *has* to be a reason—if there was no car crash, the crash sits in the inner world. The rare patient will come to therapy having a sense of this from the start: "I know that my depersonalization is a retreat. It's comfortable and safe, and I feel scared without it." A fundamental task of psychotherapy is to help patients understand the fear, the crash, and the alternative.

Unreality connotes escape from reality—not cognitive reality (DDD is not a psychosis) but rather experienced and felt reality, which has been relinquished because it is too much to bear. Schilder emphasized the negation of experiencing inherent to depersonalization—defensively, genuine experiencing is replaced by heightened and detached self-observation.[15] Ambrosino echoed this negation of self-experiencing: "In the explanation of DP there does appear to be a relationship between the degree of DP and the investment of self-experiencing" (p. 115).[16]

Depersonalization connotes a loss of personhood. The renowned pediatrician and psychoanalyst Donald Winnicott wrote about *personalization* in his essay "Basis for self in body," published in 1972, one year after his death:[17]

> I adopted the term "personalisation" as a kind of positive form of depersonalisation, which is a term that has been used and discussed fairly fully. Various meanings are given to the word "depersonalisation," but on the whole they involve the child's or the patient's loss of contact with the body and body functioning, and this implies the existence of some other aspect of the personality. The term "personalisation" was intended to draw attention to the fact that the in-dwelling of this other part of the personality in the body, and a firm link between whatever is there which we call psyche, in developmental terms represents an achievement in health. (p. 261)

Winnicott appears to be telling us that in the depersonalized person, one can find what is personalized and real, the psyche, "in-dwelling" in the body. He linked this phenomenon to the mother's failing to merge her baby's body and psyche into a whole, live being. One can readily imagine how in this scenario, the body speaks for the psyche while the mind can be hard to find. And, in fact, for those with DDD the body often speaks more clearly than the thoughts of the mind. The therapist can see the fear in the body's posture, in the staring or averted gaze, even when the patient does not seem aware of it. Personalization is not a safe enough way of being for a person who needs to relinquish the self, or they wouldn't do so—it's the ultimate price to pay. Perhaps it is the reason why so many people with DDD are prone to make the point that they would prefer any other of a long list of mental or physical ailments. Personalization has also been abandoned simply because it is not a safe enough way to exist.

The depersonalized person has trouble knowing (not through thinking but through felt experiencing) who they really are, what makes them tick, and what ails them. They have sacrificed the dangers and gratifications of genuine aliveness for the safe but dreadful deadness of non-being. Personhood may have been reasonably well established and come under unusual attack; more often it was quite tenuous to begin with. To be a person embedded in an experiencing and experienced self implies a reasonable autobiographical narrative, a story by the person about the self along the lines of "who I really am." This can be a dangerous proposition in DDD, where fear-driven compromise with confusion about "Me" is fighting to take the place of felt reality.

Along these lines, in DDD psychotherapy *unreality* and *depersonalization* often take the form of uncertainty, doubt, and confusion over what the patient has experienced, and is experiencing, in their lives. The *content* of the unreality and depersonalization varies from person to person. Ben could not dare to know that he felt emotionally used by his now-deceased mother and resented her tremendously for it. Noah had little room for feelings and could not accommodate the complexities of his ambivalence toward both his parents. Aisha's personhood lacked the entitlement and agency to pick and choose between wanted and unwanted intrusions on her being. David, very much à la Winnicott, had lost his psyche from the start, only to be found safely dwelling within the cocoon of his extreme isolation and his intense fantasy life. And Haru could not bear to know all that he felt about others who needed too much from him and gave too little in return.

Great confusion and uncertainty surrounding one's experienced, felt reality, one that is not known with emotional conviction, is depersonalizing. As humans, we tend to know when we experience something as "real" because we have the emotional conviction—in the moment, anyway; the self is not static, and neither is external reality. But in the depersonalized person, powerful psychic forces are operating against experiencing and emotional processing. Depersonalization, ultimately, is a mental escape from fully experiencing one's own reality. It is a tremendous psychic price to pay, as German psychoanalyst Karen Horney succinctly put it: "In terms of the devil's pact, the abandoning of self corresponds to the selling of one's soul.

In psychiatric terms we call it the 'alienation from self.' This latter term is applied chiefly to those extreme conditions in which people lose their feeling of identity, as in amnesias and depersonalizations, etc." (p. 155)[9] (the extreme conditions she was referring to were dissociative conditions). In contemporary times, psychologist Diana Fosha has elegantly elaborated the quality of the unintegrated, dissociative, core self-experience, in terms of the relative absence of "coherence, vitality, energy, and/or subjective truth" (p. 496).[18]

When conviction about one's felt and experienced reality is compromised and sacrificed enough, dpdr may set in, grow, and fester. Conversely, in those who for a long time and for many reasons had to unwittingly compromise with depersonalization, more "real" experiences can be a terrifying in their own right. Can one dare to trust an awakening, and will one be able to bear it? As such it is not surprising that in the therapy process, newly found experiencing and the clarity of genuine reality can, in the moment, be depersonalizing in its own right. The self is *shifting* and the process is scary, triggering the usual protection. However, the psychotherapy process is growth-promoting and headed in the direction of self-actualization. As newly found realities become safer, gratifying, and self-defining, the depersonalization that was masking them is no longer necessary.

Childhood Trauma and the Fear of Knowing

As we discussed in earlier chapters, emotional maltreatment is very common in DDD, and has even been found to predict dpdr severity. It comes in two forms, neglect and abuse; either or both may be present in a patient's history. Emotional maltreatment is a little trickier than physical or sexual abuse because where to draw the line is blurrier; there is no such thing as a perfect parent. But no one knows that line better than the subject who experienced it. As Winnicott told us, a parent can only hope and strive to be "good enough." When a parent is more seriously and consistently compromised as a caregiver, parent/child matches or mismatches, gender, changing circumstances in the parent's life, and any other extraneous factors can attenuate or magnify the damaging impact of emotional maltreatment. The same goes for when both parents are emotionally ill-equipped, or when there are no other significant adults in a child's life to come to the rescue. Other types of maltreatment *do* occur in DDD, including physical neglect, physical abuse, and sexual abuse—nearly two-thirds of patients reported at least one *clinically significant* maltreatment category on the Childhood Trauma Questionnaire (Chapter 7).

Emotional maltreatment is ubiquitous across numerous psychiatric disorders; it constitutes a broad vulnerability factor, which interacts both with biological dispositions (normative dissociation, alexithymia, temperament, heritable psychiatric syndromes) and with other life events in shaping a child's trajectory. In this sense and given the established role of emotional maltreatment in the genesis of DDD, a more focused question related to the disorder has to do with specific ingredients of the maltreatment, as well as how it is processed by the particular child.

There are no research studies providing an in-depth examination of emotional maltreatment in DDD compared to other psychiatric disorders. One study compared childhood trauma in DDD and major depression (Chapter 7) and reported comparably elevated rates of emotional abuse and neglect in the two, but the quantitative nature of the Childhood Trauma Questionnaire provided no qualitative information.[19] We've already described some of the characteristics of emotional abuse in DDD, which were obtained by a qualitative trauma interview in another study (Chapter 7).[20] It starts early in life, around age five, and involves both parents in about half of patients. And it is frequent and severe enough to create a dangerous and damaging emotional environment, wherein a child prone to dissociation may well begin to emotionally detach out of fright long before the clinical symptoms set in. Hence what we often see in clinical practice with DDD patients: some version of "nothing bad really happened," somewhere on the border of the real and the unreal.

Emotional neglect by a parent involves a diminished recognition of the child. By not mirroring, attending to, being interested in, or fostering a child's needs, wants, and unique individuality, these are invalidated, and the child's realness is squelched. This erasure can be especially damaging when a child has not had the corrective opportunity to experience an alternate reality from another caregiver or interested adult. The child may never know their own feelings well enough, especially if they have some innate difficulty with identifying them (primary alexithymia). They may have to safeguard them from others, trivialize, or sacrifice them (secondary alexithymia), and come to rely more on thinking their way through life. At its worse, and this is not unusual in DDD, the patient may seemingly have no clue that they grew up emotionally deprived—after all, omissions (neglect) are harder for any child to know than commissions (abuse).

What is unique to a patient with DDD is the tenacious confusion and emotional uncertainty surrounding the experiences of their childhood, above and beyond the emotional maltreatment itself. There is a different feel quality to a person who more or less knows things about their past with emotional conviction, albeit ambivalently, or painfully. A person who is very confused about what they experienced and felt does not have the mental "privilege" of knowing, and using that knowledge to navigate life. They are starting at a different and more difficult place (i.e., what did I really experience?). The protective function of dissociation against unbearable reality is, in and of itself, derealizing.

The childhood trauma found in DDD is often associated with a fearful attachment style[21] (Chapter 7), suggesting that parental emotional ineptitudes are at play well before the age of five and shape the child's earliest way of relating to others. As with emotional maltreatment, about half of DDD patients have fearful attachment—the numbers are telling. Relational fear is fear without an easy solution, as neither closeness nor distance engenders safety and comfort. The psychotherapy of a person with DDD therefore has to be "attachment-informed."[22] Fearful attachment plays out in the therapeutic relationship, alongside the emotional processing of traumatic experiences. Recounting and processing pockets of trauma often stirs up dpdr, not only because the trauma is painful and overwhelming to explore, but also because the patient is prone to feel alone with it as they always did, despite the therapist's presence and engagement. The aloneness is frightening and depersonalizing in its own right, and it can take time to build the relational trust that the patient very much needs to go down the path of their history more safely.

As early experiences are woven in with current life struggles and conflicts, a DDD patient comes to feel that the endeavor is meaningful and can help them in the present lives. The ways in which partners, friends, or bosses are experienced in terms of being similar to the parental imagoes, and can consequently elicit similar depersonalizing experiences, begins to make more sense. This may occur because people tend to find others akin to those who colored their past and unwittingly repeat patterns, or because fear and mistrust is triggered from the past and has no rightful place in the present, or some combination of both. A person with DDD comes to realize that closeness and intimacy dissociates them, and that they distance themselves or push others away often without knowing that they are doing so. At the same time, they come to know that experiences of aloneness may dissociate them as well, because they too are frightening. As patients become more aware of the fear-driven oscillations in how they relate to other people, and to their therapist, they begin to better regulate the relational experience in ways that can accommodate all the feelings involved and hence be less dissociating. As the fright of relating subsides so does the depersonalization, and space is created for more genuine personalization.

Alexithymia and Affect Phobia

Many people with DDD have clinically relevant alexithymia (Chapter 7), moderately or highly elevated. Sometimes it can be striking. Andrew was a patient who had pretty much three words for describing feelings when he started therapy: fine, good, and interesting. Such a constricted vocabulary fails to capture the complex and nuanced feelings of human beings; it is vague, general, and of little communicative value. Yet, it was all Andrew was capable of verbalizing, and his therapist wondered whether he had trouble with describing feelings, or couldn't sense them in the first place. Regardless, Andrew conveyed a strong need to perceive all experiences as at least OK or better, though sometimes he had to reluctantly acknowledge this was not so—apparently, negative feelings were intolerable.

There are two aspects to alexithymia, difficulty sensing feelings versus difficulty describing feelings—the two are related yet distinct. The less one internally perceives, the less one can put into words for oneself or share with others. The former may have more to do with biology and preverbal attachment trauma, the latter more with maltreatment and sociocultural expectations, but it's not clear-cut. Both components are explored and addressed in therapy. It may take more time and therapeutic work to help a patient begin to *identify* what they are feeling. Sometimes sensations only register as such, unattached to feeling (pit in the stomach, weight in the chest, and so on). Other times they register but cannot easily be translated into a rich emotional vocabulary. And at times, the vocabulary is richer on the inside, but is guardedly unshared. A patient may have learned from early life experiences that it is in vain to share—not only may they not be heard or understood, but things might even backfire.

It can be very hard for the adult DDD patient to grasp that expressing oneself is not simply about the other person understanding or agreeing, but about the genuineness of the self. A sense of dullness and dread is what patients and clinicians alike sometimes experience early on in a DDD treatment—and it is likely that other people in the patient's life feel it too. Affectless narrative needs to come to life and coming to know one's emotional world takes time—probably where the traditional psychoanalytic take of longer treatments and resistance to psychotherapy originates. At the same time, DDD alexithymia tells us that cognitive-behavioral therapy (CBT) may be barking up the wrong tree: it can help the cognitions and behaviors that are associated with DDD and exacerbate its course, but it is off target given the primacy of working with feelings in a condition characterized by emotional processing difficulties. Perhaps this is why the only treatment study of DDD that involved CBT (discussed in previous chapter) was only modestly helpful.

Alexithymia also helps explain why emotional or other maltreatment that may otherwise have been more fully processed earlier on is experienced by the DDD patient in a confused and unreal way. Alexithymia also helps us appreciate why adulthood stressors (Chapter 7) that are more ordinary than extraordinary, traumatic for some but not for others, have the potential to destabilize the self in a major way—emotional processing is already compromised, and there is a lot of emotional baggage. The diminished capacity to emotionally process adversity, from birth through adulthood, leaves those with alexithymia more vulnerable from the very beginning, and ongoingly in life. It is healthier to have an experiencing self, no matter how troubled or untroubled, than not. At some point the scale tips.

The secondary alexithymia that may accompany the hypoemotionality of dpdr may be yet another piece, and a further challenge once a patient is deep into the condition, but it's clearly not the only culprit. Though a patient may be inclined to attribute the emotional vacuum to the hypoemotionality of their depersonalized state, the real culprit likely is the alexithymia that was present way before the symptoms set in, compounded by attachment and maltreatment trauma. Secondary DDD-related alexithymia may also be at work, yet the flavor of a DDD patient who does have emotional language, even if the feelings themselves are blunted, is very different from a patient with constricted language devoid of feelings.

In psychotherapy it is apparent early on when very little feeling is expressed or discussed. The therapist may then gently but persistently encourage a patient to attach feelings to whatever they may be talking about, no matter how important or trivial. At times this process can be painstaking for patient and therapist alike, and can take a lot of time and work. Alexithymia is fertile breeding ground for depersonalization; experiences cannot be processed without their accompanying emotions, and unprocessed experiences can eventually lead to dpdr in those who've had enough negative experiences, coupled with a dissociation-proneness: patients eventually come to understand this.

There are various ways in which a patient in therapy is helped to hone in on the quality, intensity, and nuances of their emotional experiences. Psychoeducation (learning about the nature of feelings) is quite useful. Feelings are detailed, specific, and complex; often more than one is present, and they can be contradictory since they may represent conflicting aspects of one's experience. Feeling charts and wheels can be engaging and informative for some, helping a patient become more familiar with, and use, a large array of feelings on their own time. Daily feeling diaries may be appealing to some patients: a brief daily vignette can be recorded, with a focus on the emotional experience of the selected happening. The therapist might suggest what the patient may be feeling, based on what they are intuiting given their knowledge and understanding of the patient, and may offer feeling options for the patient to consider, modify, refine, or reject. This is a tentative and respectful process, recognizing that we can never fully know another's subjectivity. Clues about feeling states can be glimpsed from the totality of the context within which they are embedded—their associated bodily sensations, thoughts, behaviors, and situations in which they were stirred up.

For a patient who has more of a sense for what they are feeling inside but has trouble communicating it, the meanings of the trouble can be uncovered and understood. When there is a reluctance to share, the fears behind the reluctance are very helpful for the patient to explore; they are likely the same fears experienced in their other meaningful relationships. Often the fear is related to trauma and to fearful attachment, to a historical expectation that one's feelings will not be heard and recognized, but rather will somehow be bulldozed, attacked, belittled, ridiculed, ignored, or replaced with more "appropriate" ones.

When accessing and processing emotions is a challenge to begin with, emotions become an easier venue for defensive compromises to inner struggles, which don't work very well. Leigh McCullough, an American psychotherapist and researcher, used the term "affect phobia" to designate the fear of emotions that a person may be experiencing.[23] She described triangles of conflict, whereby one feeling is used defensively (and unconsciously) against another, more dreaded one. For example, some people are more comfortable with sadness than anger, others the reverse. Take a parent who could be comforting if the child was sad, but distanced or counterattacked when the child got angry—or, conversely, a parent who enjoyed the feistiness of protest but crumbled with the child's expressions of sadness. Understandably, the former once-child is more comfortable with sadness, the latter with anger. And then along comes a situation, like many, that requires both feelings to process and move on, such as Ben's story of depersonalization. A person with alexithymia is more likely to have an "either/or" feeling experience. The complexity of knowing and integrating the richness and contradiction of feelings is more challenging.

As a patient becomes more curious and comfortable with identifying, experiencing, and sharing feelings, the patient and the therapist alike begin to have the uncanny experience that the treatment is coming to life—lack of emotion has a deadening effect on all involved. The patient begins to learn that the world of emotions is very helpful in navigating their experiences. And through having shared, mutual emotional experiences with the therapist, the patient emotionally learns that unlike the parental imago, there are others who care about, can tolerate, and even enjoy their emotional experiences, no matter how painful, complicated, or distasteful these might seem to be. Depersonalization becomes less necessary when emotional processing happens. And beyond the "safe" therapist, the patient becomes bolder in knowing and sharing feelings with other important people in their lives, which in turn helps them experience a greater richness and genuineness in their relationships.

Adolescence and Early Adulthood Identity Struggles

Self and identity are complicated enough to grasp in their own right—though related, they are not the same. Identity has to do with the more stable and enduring perceptions of who one is, as a person and in the culture and world in which they're embedded. Psychologist Erik Erikson was rooted in Freudian theory but expanded our thinking with his "stage theory of psychosocial development," taking note of defining developmental tasks that occur *after* early childhood, and throughout the lifespan. He saw identity as a "fundamental organizing principal which develops constantly throughout the lifespan" and involves the experiences, relationships, memories, beliefs and values, and ambitions that constitute a person's subjective sense of self.

In the classic book *Childhood and Society*, written in 1950, Erikson described adolescence as the life stage whose major developmental task *centers on identity versus confusion*.[24] Identity formation begins in very early life, starts to consolidate in adolescence, and is further developed and defined into "early" adulthood (age 18 to 25 or so). Also referred to as "emerging" or "young" adulthood, this life period is critically important for attaining a cohesive-enough sense of self that feels like a "Me."

Concurrent with Erikson's developmental stage theory, Robert J. Havighurst, a renaissance man of the 1900s—a physicist, researcher, educator, civil rights activist, and prolific writer—in 1948 developed a theory of the different developmental tasks applicable to different age periods.[25] The developmental tasks of adolescence and early adulthood, according to Havighurst, who originally divided them a little too neatly before and after age 18, included acceptance of one's body, masculine/feminine roles, emotional stability and autonomy from parents, close peer friendships, professional preparation and pursuit, a personal moral code and social responsibility, intimacy and stable partnerships, social group affiliations, and contemplation of a family of one's own. It is a lot, indeed, and it is no wonder that so many young adults are struggling in today's world.

Yet, there is some fundamental truth to the importance of a solid-enough adolescent and young adult identity. A 2007 longitudinal study tested Havighurst's model in boys/men and girls/women from the age of 14 to 23, assessed six times over the one-decade time period.[26] The study found support both for the interrelatedness and progressive attainment of these tasks over the 10 years, and for meaningful links between developmental achievements and general symptomatology. It was not all smooth sailing, and it was clear that the timeframe for young adulthood has expanded over recent decades, and that self-esteem is not readily predictable. Yet, developmental achievements did matter: higher developmental status and lower symptomatology were consistently associated, both concurrently and longitudinally.

DDD has an average age of onset in adolescence or late adolescence, and so the looming developmental challenges unique to this age group are often at play in the genesis of the disorder and may be a major focus and part of the psychotherapy, especially in patients who seek help in this age group. Erik Erikson saw "confusion" as the alternative to identity—and DDD immediately jumps to mind. Compromise with confusion as a semi-successful adaptation in earlier life, as we discussed in the maltreatment section, can start to falter during the important transition to adulthood, in which room for confusion and uncertainty lessens. There are rising psychological and sociocultural expectations, even demands, for clarity regarding values, goals, plans, work, relationships, and the like.

Guralnik and Simeon highlighted that in DDD, as a quintessential pathology of personhood, it is crucial, in some patients at least, to consider the interface with the larger context of culture, and the interplay between recognition and interpellation forces.[27] Richard Chefetz, a dissociation clinician and theorist, proposed that societal forces are more relevant to maintaining and perpetuating dpdr rather than causing it; the dpdr is more likely to be rooted in the terror of earlier family dynamics, which later symbolically plays out in the realm of social discourse.[28] This matter need not be an either/or, and there may be situations in which sociocultural pressures were put on a child so early in life through the parents' own unprocessed sociocultural struggles that the two are not distinguishable. Along these lines, LaMothe broadly defined personalization as "diverse forms of recognizing the other as a unique, responsive, inviolable, and valued subject, all of which are contingent upon community," similarly at play in the personalization of a child through "good enough" parenting and the personalization of all individuals who truly belong to and are supported by a community (p. 271).[29]

Not surprisingly, a stabler and stronger sense of identity is protective against mental illness in general, and DDD in particular; conversely, identity confusion is a vulnerability. It is strikingly common to see patients whose DDD started in their senior year of high school, their first year of college, their senior year of college, or the first year of their post-college career. These transitions activate the nascent conflicts and struggles subsuming tenuous and shaky identity formation, and the earlier compromises that offered some stability into high school begin to fall apart.

Young adults with DDD, like many young adults, unwittingly minimize the relevance, power, and difficulty of these transitions. They often intellectually emphasize how normative these transitions are meant to be, and how all their peers and friends are navigating them seemingly without difficulty. Compounding things, people in this age group may be reluctant to share their troubling experiences with others, and many colleges pay inadequate attention to mental health and illness. Before deeper exploration, therapy can help in dispelling the myth of a seamless transition into adulthood, one perpetuated by the continuing stigma surrounding mental illness that the COVID pandemic has tragically begun to shake up. The young adult in therapy can be helped to emotionally recognize how life-changing, big, and difficult these transitions are, doing away with stereotypes and stigmas and opening up space for a more *personalized* exploration.

Worrying and Obsessing: Functions and Meanings

In the previous chapter on cognitive-behavioral approaches to catastrophic thinking and obsessional ruminating we covered specific techniques for tackling these symptoms. But worrying and obsessing serve additional functions—when the mind is possessed and consumed by them, there is little mental space left to attend to anything else. In this way, typically outside a patient's awareness, the psychic forces that precipitated dpdr in the first place remain unknown. If patient and therapist cannot find a way to put aside the worry and obsessing in sessions, for some of the time anyway, and broach the deeper underlying issues, these will remain nascent and will likely continue to erupt despite some symptomatic improvement with CBT or medication.

Early on it may be difficult or, at times, nearly impossible to take this angle in an exploratory psychotherapy, if a patient is not in a state of mind to hear about it or bear it. When immediate symptom relief is center stage in those who present more acutely, even brief lapses of *remembering that there is a person behind the symptoms* can counteract the depersonalized state and be grounding. Talk of the person behind the symptoms can feel like a respite at times, a revelation at others, or an irritating distraction from dpdr-focused anxiety. At some point the anxiety symptoms will predictably improve, whether it be with medication, some CBT or mindfulness-based techniques, or simply the comfort and hope that starting psychotherapy often engenders. There may even be a resolution of the immediate crisis that led the patient to seek treatment at a particular point in time. As a person settles into the new therapy and begins to feel more trusting and allied with the therapist, they become more curious and engaged in the bigger picture of who they are and what ails them.

A more specific theme to all the worrying and obsessing in DDD is the *illusion of control* that they are in the service of. It is as if it helps to get a better grip on the symptoms, investigate them leaving no stone unturned, and magically solve them. This is, of course, not so. CBT is based on the premise that the anxiety only fuels the dpdr, and any exploratory psychotherapy can help drive this point home as well—even as it eclectically adopts some techniques that are useful for the patient to manage the symptoms. But there may be an additional matter to explore, such as whether a patient's personality, vulnerabilities, past traumas, and current life circumstances are feeding into the worrying and obsessing. Those prone to fearfulness or perfectionism, those who are intolerant of uncertainty, those who are overly invested in quick results, or those who are going through turbulent life events may feel even more out-of-control and destabilized by the onset of dpdr. It is helpful to contextualize the overwhelmingness of the dpdr in these ways, lessening the symptoms' power over the person. The focus can begin to shift from the symptoms to other areas of the patient's experience, to how the patient may have started to feel less in control, more vulnerable and at sea, lost in an inner world that was getting harder to navigate, *before* the dpdr set in.

Despite the rather predictable repertory to the kinds of dpdr-focused anxieties that plague those with DDD, the *content* of these anxieties is still useful to explore, looking for psychodynamic clues to better under- stand their terrifying grip on the person. Marianne, a young woman with DDD, endlessly ruminated about existence and infinity whenever her dpdr intensified—or vice versa. She was neither a philosopher nor a physicist, so the question arose: Why was she so caught up with existence? Why turn to nihilism? It turned out that her parents had divorced when she was seven and she spent designated nights with her father, who was an astronomy pro- fessor and a very emotionally unavailable man. When Marianne lay sleep- less in bed at night fearing the dark and the void, her father would come to her room, but could only offer, in his usual factual voice, wisdoms about the universe: things about the nature of dark and light, the warping of time, or what happens to consciousness after the body dies. Such words were hardly comforting to a young, though very bright, girl. They simply represented the dreadful void of emotional absence, and left Marianne alone in the same fear as before her dad came to the room to comfort her. Her existential ruminations symbolized the terror that no one would be there for her when she was truly in desperate need, as she now was in her adult life when she sought out therapy.

DDD Triggered by Drugs: Does Psychodynamic Therapy Make Sense?

This question can sometimes be a tricky one, but not as tricky as it may sound at first. Take, for example, the case of a seemingly well-adjusted young adult who was doing well in the major areas of life, vaped marijuana for the third time, and entered chronic dpdr. He is convinced this was a chemical event, and terribly bad luck, and doubts that there is anything deeper to discover. He may appear to be making a good point. It is for the therapist to conduct an open-minded exploration of whether more could be at play. Very often, this is the case. According to the chemical argument (see Chapter 6), only particular drugs induce DDD, and therefore something must be involved having to do with the chemical nature of those drugs. On the other hand, the culprit drugs have mind-altering properties (hallucinogens, marijuana, salvia, MDMA, ketamine) and overwhelmingly induce "bad trips" when associated with the onset of dpdr. Opiates and cocaine, for example, are generally euphoric and do not trigger dpdr. A bad trip, in and of itself, can be so terrifying for many, especially the extreme case where a person literally believes that they have died, that that fact alone could conceivably trigger a depersonalization episode.

The psychodynamic question, which is well worth entertaining and engaging a patient's curiosity, is whether something with *meaningful*, personal content might have been experienced during the high. It is quite conceivable that a well-buried inner struggle rose to the surface, and was experienced in such a powerful live way that it could not be buried once the intoxication cleared. Take, for example, a closeted young man who has known from a very young age that he was attracted to boys yet cruised through the first two years of college dating women and pretending to himself that he like them well enough—until the fateful night he smoked pot with his buddies, one of whom was openly and comfortably gay. During the bad trip he was convinced that his gay friend was coming on to him, felt excited and horrified, and ran for his life out of the fraternity. The floodgates had opened.

A person's attribution of DDD solely to a drug always needs to be examined closely, and a patient's history is always more complicated than we initially know. It often is the case that the drug was one of several precipitating events over a brief, or more extended, period of escalating dpdr. For reasons to be understood, it's the *one* event that the patient has preferentially fixated on— yet other powerful forces may have been at play, unknown to the person starting therapy. In another scenario, a briefer dpdr episode, or episodes, had occurred before the drug-induced "big" one: What could that mean? Exploration of the earlier episodes can be revealing: if they were precipitated by a particular conflict or state of mind, something akin could be at work now, intensified by the drug's influence.

Take a 33-year-old woman eager to have children who had been struggling over whether to give her undecided boyfriend of seven years a marriage ultimatum, or just walk away. At moments of peak crisis she had depersonalized for a few hours on three occasions, she told her new therapist. Then the patient and her boyfriend smoked pot together one night, she experienced a heightened state of blissful intimacy though her dilemma had not changed, and she woke up intensely depersonalized the next morning. This time it lasted, and two months later she sought out the therapist.

Patients sometimes ask, "Is it possible that if I hadn't smoked weed I would *never* have become depersonalized?" Yes, anything is possible—we don't understand the brain enough to say otherwise. Even in the disorder of schizophrenia, where magnitudes more is known, the relationship of marijuana use to emerging psychosis has yet to be figured out. The brain and the mind are anything but static, so a more helpful way to think about this question is that the future is not scripted: early illness is a process in the making, and early treatment may help to change the course. A suffering person wants to do everything they can to help themselves and tackle a problem from all possible angles. A course of exploratory psychotherapy will help to do that.

Concluding Remarks

Exit from subjectively experiencing reality, in the form of depersonalization, happens when already compromised self-experiencing and emotionally unprocessed experience hit a tipping point. This fits with the time course and progression of both transient dpdr and DDD. There may be earlier episodes, brief and self-contained, processed and resolved outside a person's conscious efforts; they happen frequently in the "general population" and don't reach the magnitude of a disorder. But unprocessed experiences can only accumulate over time. And on the other side of the fence of unprocessed self-experience sits a dissociative propensity, at play all along in more and less adaptive ways, now inviting a pathological rescue exit. The breaking point may be gradual or sudden, and the self no longer feels like "Me."

Because emotional processing is key to self-experiencing, alexithymia is an important and common trait and state vulnerability in DDD, whether more primary or secondary, regardless of its origins in biology, attachment disturbances, maltreatment, or all of the above. Other vulnerabilities are probably involved as well, such as a fearful inhibited temperament or a familial risk for anxiety, fueling fearful and anxious responses to life events in general, and to adversities in particular, from early on in life.

Though physical or sexual traumas are encountered in a significant minority of those with DDD and cannot be overlooked, parental emotional unavailability and mistreatment from a very young age are the bread and butter of the condition, likely from the very start of life in those with fearful, or even preoccupied, attachment. Emotional and other traumas are bound to be particularly challenging for children who have difficulty sensing and processing their feelings. It makes it much harder to navigate the world of emotions and adversities, to mentalize and to make meaning of one's experiences, and to inhabit a story of who one is, a Me, that feels real. Personalization and realization have been compromised and tenuous all along.

Many proverbs are wise, but there may be no proverb more inaccurate and flat-out wrong than "sticks and stones may break my bones, but words can never hurt me." The characteristics and qualities of the emotional traumas paint a DDD picture that, at its worse, involved both parents, in different but complementary and colluding ways, chronically and relentlessly, leaving a child with little room for emotional respite or psychological repair. It is important to keep in mind that trauma is never about the "magnitude" of the events alone, no matter how major. Even in soldiers who face combat, about one-third develop PTSD. Trauma is not a competition over how bad it was, but foremost and solely in the eye of the beholder who lived it, their vulnerabilities as well as their strengths and resilience. Magnitude is only relevant, and relative, to the person who must contend with it, and heal.

Different patients with DDD will respond to psychodynamic psychotherapy differently, in terms of pace, duration, and change, as happens in any psychotherapy. It is generally fair and true to say that the earlier a patient seeks treatment, and the longer they stick it out, the better the outcome. Some inner struggles can be more deeply rooted and tenacious than others, and depersonalization itself makes it harder for the treatment to be personal, at first. It is also fair to say, based on clinicians' experience with DDD, that when dpdr is very chronic over many years, or continuous without symptom-free time periods, or at a baseline flatline of sorts with little fluctuation, the therapy can be more challenging and arduous. Regardless, psychological troubles and psychiatric conditions alike have a way of progressing and worsening, and making life more and more difficult, when left untreated. There is no better path to help and healing than exploratory psychodynamic psychotherapy, especially when other interventions have not sufficed, as is often the case.

14

Digital Depersonalization

We shape our tools, and thereafter our tools shape us.
—Marshall McLuhan

Among its many treasures, Boston's Museum of Fine Arts houses one of the largest and most intriguing works by the post-Impressionist Paul Gauguin. The massive oil on canvas depicting scenes of daily life among the Tahitians has been the subject of many interpretations since it was created in 1897–1898. An infant in one corner and a dying old woman in the other hint at the endless cycle of life and death. Left of center, a blue idol alludes to faith in a reality beyond what's depicted elsewhere on the canvas. Allegedly created during a deep psychological crisis, what makes the painting stand out, aside from its size, is its title. Scrawled in the upper left corner is the painting's title: *D'où venons-nous? Que sommes-nous? Où allons-nous?* (Where Do We Come From? What Are We? Where Are We Going?).

This work was Gauguin's response to a changing world—an unspoiled, primitive culture infiltrated by French colonization and corrupted by syphilis and other "Western" maladies. The title suggests a pause amid life's struggles and routines to question its very purpose, not only for the Tahitians but the French as well. Just as in Gauguin's Tahiti, societal changes and technological advances affect the individual. During the century that followed, the world would evolve in ways that Gauguin, let alone Maori natives, could barely begin to imagine.

Tribal cultures have traditionally placed the group above the individual. "Civilized" cultures, in Gauguin's time and today, place a premium on the individual over the group. The Industrial Revolution, and technology that quickly evolved from the steam engine to the smartphone, most often originated in the minds of individuals with imaginative brains

Feeling Unreal. Second Edition. Daphne Simeon and Jeffrey Abugel, Oxford University Press. © Oxford University Press 2023. DOI: 10.1093/oso/9780197622445.003.0014

and formidable egos. Where personhood reigns, *depersonalization* may emerge. Back in Europe, this phenomenon did not go unnoticed by *fin de siècle* doctors and philosophers. Dugas, Krishaber, Janet, and others were exploring states of detachment and unreality that often included excessive rumination about what Gauguin had inscribed. By way of Amiel's *Journal Intime*, the term *depersonalization* entered the vocabulary of psychologists and philosophers alike.

Depersonalization/derealization disorder (DDD) remained an obscure syndrome through much of the twentieth century. The medical literature was limited to observations in early scholarly articles. As relics of the past, these were sometimes difficult to locate, even for medical professionals. Armed with only their own symptoms, patients had little means of learning about depersonalization/derealization (dpdr), and even less chance of having it properly diagnosed and treated.

The birth of the internet changed all that forever. Almost from the outset, simple websites like the Netherlands-based "Unreal" quickly appeared, along with discussion groups and the online publication of whatever clinical papers could be found. The floodgates opened as young people posted their personal stories, which often included triggers that had barely been recognized in the past—marijuana, Ecstasy, ketamine, and other substances.

In time, the number of websites, discussion groups, Facebook pages, and tweets exploded to what it is today. Terminology relegated to the *Diagnostic and Statistical Manual of Mental Disorders* (*DSM*) and other scholarly references now became part of a kind of collective consciousness embodied by the internet. Even if the term *depersonalization* was unfamiliar, an online user could easily stumble across it by simply describing their symptoms. While the internet made information about depersonalization accessible to the general public, it also fostered a profusion of misinformation, self-help programs, and online gurus promising to put an end to this baffling condition. Newcomers found it difficult to sort through the new material in search of the truth.

The first edition of *Feeling Unreal*, published in 2006, helped unmuddy the waters. Dpdr subsequently appeared in movies, music videos, radio discussions, social media, and mainstream print media. But as feelings of unreality and loss of the "usual, expected sense of self" came as close as it had ever been to being a mainstream topic, so did a closer look at the medium through which this new depersonalization community was able to emerge.

Social media gave birth to the phenomenon of self-designed online identities. Just as it had transpired between pen pals and members of "lonely hearts" clubs in years past, participants could exaggerate their virtues and eliminate their flaws (hiding the truth and then being found out was a staple of black-and-white sitcoms). The internet was dramatically different from the classifieds, however: it sped things up, and false selves could be presented and edited indefinitely. For some, cyber life replaced real life, as friends, fans, followers, and other electronic beings provided a constant flow of positive reinforcement usually unavailable in the non-virtual world. A brave new cyber world unfolded with an entire generation of millennials and Gen Zs who had never experienced life without the internet or a cellphone. Handheld devices became an appendage for many, particularly young people, and from their perspective they were as necessary as hands or feet.

Sherry Turkle, clinical psychologist and professor of social studies of science at the Massachusetts Institute of Technology, has long been a vocal critic of social media and its effects on the individual self. In her book *Alone Together,* she writes: "The technology has become like a phantom limb, it is so much a part of them. These young people are among the first to grow up with an expectation of continuous connection: always on, and always on them. And they are among the first to grow up not necessarily thinking of simulation as second best. All of this makes them fluent with technology but brings a set of new insecurities" (p. 17).[1]

Inevitably, studies about the effects of technology on the brain, personality, and self-image would emerge. Could electronic identities have some effect on real-life identities, away from the computer or phone? Can people become addicted to the internet, Instagram, Facebook, or other apps? Are people with certain mental disorders more prone to relying on their cyber identities? To the timeless debate about the false self and the true self, a third party was added—the digital self.

The Self as a Network

In recent years, psychologists, sociologists, and media pundits have scrutinized cyber life and its effects on the individual. The terminology of the digital world has made its way into mainstream psychology as well. In pre-internet times, the word "network" usually related to television networks. Its definition eventually broadened to include two or more computers linked together. Now its connotations may include the varied online selves presented differently to different parties. A polished professional profile presented on LinkedIn, for instance, may be very different than what is presented on Instagram or other social media (employers taking the time to explore these venues are often surprised at what they find.)

The individual self can be viewed as a network as well, according to some current thinking. Kathleen Wallace, a professor of philosophy at New York's Hofstra University, has written about the "network self" and the importance of personal and social relationships in defining the self. The "network self" comprises the various ongoing and changing components of a person's identity. This may include interacting with others as a spouse, mother, father, church member, employee, friend, or lover. We are all creatures of our times and our societies, whether we recognize it or not. The network view brings this reality to the fore by including it as part of our self-definition. Wallace observes:

> On the psychological view, a self is a personal consciousness. On the animalist view, a self is a human organism, or animal. This has tended to lead to a somewhat one-dimensional and simplified view of what a self is, leaving out social, cultural and interpersonal traits that are also distinctive of selves and are often what people would regard as central to their self-identity. Just as selves have different personal memories and self-awareness, they can have different social and interpersonal relations, cultural backgrounds, and personalities. The latter are variable in their specificity but are just as important to being a self as biology, memory and self-awareness.[2]

Whether the network self is a fresh concept or simply a repackaging of the obvious, the social connections on which it relies may be minimized or unrecognized by depersonalized individuals. However, recognizing their existence can come into play as part of the path to healing. One former DDD sufferer put it this way:

> The idea of a network-self kind of reinforced what I began to realize on my own as I felt better. I realized that I spent too much time clinging to a false cyber world. I tried to look at the *real* elements that made up my life—my boyfriend, my interest in fashion, continuing education, even my car—and little by little I regained interest in these different aspects of my life. I tried to

eliminate the digital crutches I had relied on and find joy in the *real* things that helped me define myself. I guess when I put them all together, they made up "me." They made up a network of "me."

Changing Brains

The last two decades have yielded not only massive expansion of technology as well as social media's power and influence, but also a flurry of outspoken critics, who, along with Turkle, point out the potential dangers of the internet, backed up by considerable research. PCs, laptops, and smartphones have affected not only our work, our daily routines, and our social interactions, but our brains as well. According to cyber critics, the onscreen barrage of ads, news snippets, hyperlinks, and tweets is negatively affecting our ability to focus and absorb the written word the way we did when it appeared exclusively in print.

In his bestselling book *The Shallows: What the Internet is Doing to Our Brains*, Nicholas Carr points out that throughout the centuries, every new means of communicating ideas has affected the wiring of our brains and how we think.[3] From Sumerian cuneiforms to Gutenberg's movable type, which fostered the sharing of texts and ideas en masse, each advance in literacy has changed society and our brains themselves. Today's technology may be having a profound effect as well—a negative effect on how we create short- and long-term memories.

"The key to memory consolidation is attentiveness," Carr writes. "The sharper the attention, the sharper the memory. The influx of competing messages that we receive whenever we go online not only overloads our working memory. It makes it much harder for our frontal lobes to concentrate our attention on any one thing. The process of memory consolidation can't even get started."[3] And, because of the plasticity of our neural pathways, Carr suggests, the more we use the web, "the more we train our brains to be distracted—to process information very quickly and very efficiently but without sustained attention" (p. 194).[3]

Neuroplasticity, the brain's ability to change and adapt, has also become a topic of increasing interest. While its implications are largely positive, there is also a downside. "The more a sufferer concentrates on his symptoms, the deeper those symptoms are etched into his neural circuits," Carr observes. "In the worst cases, the mind essentially trains itself to be sick" (p. 35).[3] Such changes in the brain reflect the experiences of depersonalized individuals for whom excessive rumination about their condition, or the existential questions that haunted Gauguin, become a primary symptom that may predate internet use. The brain gets used to a computer-generated distraction rut just as the depersonalized get stuck in a self-perpetuating rut of obsessive thinking.

"Technology is seductive when what it offers meets our human vulnerabilities," Turkle observes. "And as it turns out, we are very vulnerable indeed. We are lonely but fearful of intimacy. Digital connections and the sociable robot may offer the illusion of companionship without the demands of friendship. Our networked life allows us to hide from each other, even as we are tethered to each other. We'd rather text than talk" (p. 1).[1] A depersonalized individual is particularly vulnerable to such seductions.

Zoomed Out

As the use of Zoom and other video conferencing tools has skyrocketed in lieu of human interaction, the phenomenon of "Zoom fatigue" is drawing media attention. Cyber conferencing can be hard on the brain, according to an article by Julia Sklar in *National Geographic*.[4] The brain relies on subtle nonverbal cues and body language during in-person communication. Video chats lack these nuances, and the result is a brain tired of trying to find them. "There's a lot of research that shows we actually really struggle with this," says Andrew Franklin, Assistant Professor of Cyberpsychology at Norfolk State University. "For somebody who's really dependent on those nonverbal cues, it can be a big drain not to have them," he says.[4]

Multiperson screens magnify this exhausting problem, Sklar states: "Gallery view—where all meeting participants appear *Brady Bunch*-style—challenges the brain's central vision, forcing it to decode so many people at once that no one comes through meaningfully, not even the speaker."[4]

Some people have adjusted to these restrictions and adapted to the digital substitutions for real human life. They enjoy the efficiency of work by Skype, the convenience of Zoom, and the comfort of family gatherings by FaceTime. However, others feel suffocated by the surroundings of "false digital surrogacy." They miss the freedom and authenticity of real life with friendly handshakes and hugs. They feel lost, incomplete, and different.

A student reports, "I feel like a strange copy of me is participating in a Zoom class, while another me is watching this from the side. It is like in a dream. As if I need to wake up to get myself back."

Psychologist Elena Bezzubova, who writes a blog for *Psychology Today*, is credited with first using the term "digital depersonalization." She says:

> Virtual reality, the experience of digitally created cyberspace, is . . . considered by some enthusiasts to be a new form of consciousness. However, people with depersonalization have been long familiar with the experiences which are strikingly similar to this cyber-phenomenon. Virtual reality is a digitally generated imagery (acoustic, visual, tactile, etc.) which is nearly indistinguishable from the real reality of the objective world. Digitally built environments not only imitate reality, but are open for almost complete immersion by and active interaction with a user.[5]

Some observers feel that the world of virtual reality (VR) and headsets that transport conscious existence into an entirely different world is an even greater challenge to individual authenticity than simply being someone else online. Bezzubova believes that there are parallels between the unreal world of these simulations and the mental experiences of those living with chronic depersonalization. "Depersonalization is a virtual condition: an effectual experience of unreality that does not have a factual ground," she states (p. 94).[6]

"Virtual reality and depersonalization complement each other as mirror reflections. They are both experiences of virtuality, but directed to opposite sides. Virtual reality is the digital imagery of reality. Depersonalization (virtual unreality) is the neuronal imagery of *unreality*. Thus, virtuality is an experience that can be created by both machines and human brains. Virtual reality is 'as-if' reality; depersonalization is 'as-if' unreality" (p. 94).[6]

"The Greek word *persona* translates into English as mask," Bezzubova notes. "Avatars, selfies, memojis and animojis are translations of the persona-mask into the language of the digital world. Greek actors cover their faces with masks that fit their roles on the stage of Greek theater. Inhabitants of the digital community cover themselves with avatars and selfies to better fit their roles on the digital stage. The first digital settlements, Myspace and Facebook, became unprecedented labs of self-crafting masquerades" (p. 99).[6]

Virtual Unreality

As VR evolves from science fiction to science fact, one pertinent question arises: Can immersion in an unreal VR world induce symptoms of depersonalization and derealization in "normal" people? A 2022 study from Germany found that the answer is yes.[7] Conducted by the Department of Psychiatry at the University of Bonn, the study included 80 participants (38 female), all having normal or corrected-to-normal vision and no current psychiatric or neurological disorders. To make certain that participants were mentally healthy, a variety of assessments were utilized, including the Cambridge Depersonalization Scale, the Depersonalization Severity Scale, the Beck Depression Inventory, and others.

For both groups, the computer game *The Elder Scrolls V: Skyrim* from Bethesda Game Studios was used as the experimental intervention. *Skyrim* is a widespread action/fantasy role-playing game, with more than 30 million copies sold. It was selected not only because of its popularity but also because of its high immersiveness and VR compatibility. Regardless of their group allocation, all participants played the same entrance scene of *Skyrim*, in which the player has to flee a dragon through underground tunnels and dungeons. This scene was chosen because it induces a high level of arousal and experiential vividness, and requires no previous game experience; also its game control is sufficiently easy, according to the researchers.

The study found that participants experienced transient symptoms of depersonalization and derealization after both VR gaming and PC gaming. However, there were significantly stronger increases in dpdr experiences immediately after VR gaming, as opposed to playing the same game on a PC. In both groups, the amount of dpdr experience was considerably greater while playing than at baseline. While the study confirms an earlier finding of dpdr induction by a single VR session,[8] it documents dpdr experiences in both VR and PC gaming, stronger after VR gaming. Why PC gaming, and in particular VR gaming, induces dpdr aftereffects remains unclear. According to the authors, one intuitive explanation is that a subject just immersed in a "new virtual reality" and then thrown back into "old ordinary reality" might experience a transient predictive uncertainty as to which of the two competing reality models is the more veridical one.

One question remains: How might VR affect people already suffering from DDD? That question remains unanswered.

Power of the Pandemic

The effects of ever-changing technology on the way people think, work, and socialize will no doubt continue to provide rich material for social observers in the years ahead. Digital media create unique depersonalizing scenarios, whether through VR, internet addiction, or social media interactions that foster the creation of limitless digital selves. During the COVID-19 lockdown, digital media use increased dramatically, according to *Forbes* magazine: as early as May 2020, worldwide internet use had increased by nearly 70%, and streaming by 12%.[9] Did this dramatic change in day-to-day living have an effect on people suffering from DDD? Did it trigger the disorder in people vulnerable to it? Maybe so. Two obvious and distinct pathways may have been at play: the burnout associated with the pandemic experience, and the increased use of digital media secondary to the pandemic.

Regarding the former, studies have already documented the increased rates of dpdr associated with COVID-19 burnout. Galanis and colleagues reviewed 16 studies of nurses who worked during the pandemic in 2020.[10] Nearly 20,000 participants were examined, and the overall prevalence of depersonalization was 12.6%, approximately one in eight—surpassing that of nurses who work in traditional extremely stressful settings such as the palliative care of terminal patients. Furthermore, preexisting dissociative symptoms increased the likelihood of pandemic-related posttraumatic stress disorder (PTSD) in frontline hospital workers.[11] In groups where the pandemic has been just one of many major social stressors, such as Libyan healthcare workers, depersonalization was reported by almost half.[12]

And, as importantly, the pandemic witnessed a massive shift to virtual engagement, as Bezzubova notes:

> The pandemic has changed the balance between the real world and virtual imagery, making a person more susceptible to digital depersonalization. The pre-pandemic world of freedom of movement and human relationships has become a paradise lost. What we once experienced as a human world with optional digital interaction has now become a cyberspace with allowed doses of human interaction. For a birthday party, a physician's consult, or a meeting with a friend, we now have to go to nonexistent virtuality. There is something disturbing and depersonalizing in this twisted way of relating to yourself, others, and the world around you.[13]

Exploring the effects of social isolation further, Anna Ciaunica and colleagues conducted an online study involving 622 participants worldwide to investigate the relationship between digital media-based activities and distal social actions in influencing people's sense of self during the lockdown compared to before the pandemic.[14] The study revealed that increased use of "sedentary digital media consumption" (watching films, TV, YouTube videos, etc.) and "digital media-based activities," particularly playing computer games and participating in online social e-meetings via Zoom, Skype, and so forth, correlated with higher feelings of depersonalization. Participants who reported that the lockdown influenced their life to a greater extent also had higher occurrences of depersonalization experiences. As Ciaunica and coworkers note:

> Our findings may help tackle key questions related to the human mental well-being during a lockdown in the general population. This study suggests that increasing virtual social interactions (i.e., sedentary and screen-based) and digital activities may have negative effects in some people, by making them feel less "real" and more detached from their selves, their bodies, and others. These results point to potential risks related to an overly sedentary and hyper-digitalized life habits that may induce feelings of living in one's head, disconnected from one's body, self, and the world. (p. 15)[14]

Internet Addiction

In 2019, a study of 253 Italian young adults (52% female) aged between 18 and 25 indicated a strong relationship between problematic internet use (PIU) and preexisting conditions of negative affectivity, dismissive attachment, and dpdr symptoms.[15] The findings suggested that "excessive time spent online may combine with maladaptive personality features, insecure attachment dispositions, and difficulties in processing bodily experiences in generating PIU among young adults" (p. 447).[15] The same research group examined 364 *World of Warcraft* gamers, aged 18 to 48, and found that PIU scores were positively associated with alexithymia, a trait that is prevalent in DDD.[16]

To date, there is no consensus on how much time online actually constitutes "problematic" internet use. It has been suggested that the more time a person spends online, the higher the arousal when that person is connected. Subsequently, the interest in and arousal toward non-virtual social stimuli are lowered, leading to altered health habits and interference in the social, family, academic, or work domains. According to a study of Spanish university students, PIU can represent a maladaptive coping strategy for young individuals who display maladaptive personality traits, difficulties in integrating their internal experiences, and problems in close relationships.[17] By extension, it is possible that for some people with DDD, the internet may provide a place in which to avoid real life and escape feelings of depersonalization.

Another study, by Bernardi and Pallanti,[18] linked PIU to dissociative symptoms in a group of 50 psychiatric outpatients with mixed diagnoses, and specifically identified a strong relationship between time spent on the web and dissociative symptoms. Lastly, Schimmenti and Caretti have proposed an extreme syndrome coined "video-terminal dissociative trance" (VDT) that can result from overtly excessive internet use. VDT "may involve significant disturbances in the state of consciousness, identity, and memory, the dilution of self-awareness and self-integrity, and the replacement of the customary sense of personal identity by a new virtual identity" (p. 455).[19]

In Japan, the phenomenon of *hikikomori* has been growing since the 1970s. The disorder mainly affects adolescents or young adults who live cut off from the world, cloistered within their parents' homes, locked in their bedrooms for days, months, or even years. They refuse to communicate even with their families, use the internet profusely, and only venture out to deal with their most imperative bodily needs. Many *hikikomori* turn to the internet, and sometimes spend more than 12 hours a day in front of the computer. As a consequence, more than half of them are at risk of internet addiction, and approximately one-tenth would fit diagnostic criteria for such an addiction.[20]

The *DSM-5* now recognizes "internet gaming disorder," but PIU is not yet part of the manual. Regardless, the relationship between these two conditions and DDD has not been investigated. However, one tumblr *hikikomori* may well be expressing what is experienced by thousands of silent, isolated teens:

I feel unreal. You seem unreal. Everything seems unreal. I can't tell if you're all robots and this is some sort of *Truman Show* plot, or if you're all just machinations of my own mind. Is this some sort of simulation? I can't tell. Honestly, it's almost as if I'm in some fake, virtual reality. I constantly try to find glitches in the system to validate these thoughts. Another idea is that you wake up from a dream, into another dream. Like *Inception* but in real life.

One young woman living with her parents in Denmark has not left for house for four years, except for emergency room visits and a short stay in the hospital. A psychologist from social services visits on a periodic basis, and while Astrid hasn't been formally diagnosed with DDD, she identifies with the symptoms and is the member of several internet groups dedicated to it. Astrid's relationship with her parents is tenuous at best. "They've given up on me," she says. "I don't blame them. They've taken me to a lot of doctors who say I'm depressed, or bipolar and agoraphobic. I've tried a ton of meds but nothing helps. Every time I leave the house, or try to get somewhere in the car, I feel like I'm going to pass out. I have panic attacks and then everything seems like a dream. It doesn't clear up until I'm back in my room."

Despite her inability to deal with even the most mundane tasks of life, Astrid has created and sustained a formidable online presence. She has recorded numerous YouTube videos about everything from applying unusual makeup, to "whisper" therapies, to sensual kisses directed to the camera and hence the person on the other end, to love poems to her boyfriend. "I do tactile, sensual things," she says, "not sexual stuff." Her boyfriend visits regularly, supplementing her online presence with empathy and flesh and blood.

"She's a very special person," he says. "I know that her life isn't normal. I've tried to take her out to places but it never works." While experiencing day-to-day life as unreal, Astrid's online presence has become her primary reality. Her depersonalization predates her internet use, but internet addiction has become the anchor that grounds her very existence.

Another example illustrates the smartphone's unique role as pacifier and companion, a modern replacement for what pediatrician and psychoanalyst D. W. Winnicott defined as a "transitional object"—a child's favored plush toy or comforting baby blanket offering feelings of security.[6] One sufferer captured such a unique relationship with her phone in a poem:

My sterile and cold-blooded lover, you fillip me dawn after dawn,
sleep still in my eyes. I turn to embrace you, wrap my hand around

your solid white back. I peruse your eyes, icons lit to my pleasing,
waiting at my-beck-and-call. I touch your blue eye to awaken

my mind-game brain: I still have the IQ knack. I touch your green eye,
wildly indexing up and down: when will you and I afford glamping?

You have so many eyes, like the scallop! Sixty-two at last count,
neatly arranged around the edge of your thick core. All compete

for a teeny-wholesome-corner of my shattered mind. You ground
me so, and do not ask for much: I just pay you once-a-month.

Not quite an escort, you offer sex whenever I want, untethered.
Scallop—our morning embrace done, I'm fired to take on

the day's tedium, grateful to my 3x6 rechargeable and ever-present
bud. But really, should I be? God damn you Scallop! You're all

I have left. You're not soft melt-in-the-mouth, I can't cook you
to my pleasing. A deluded stand-in for the many eyes of regret.

Your blue eye the blues. Your green eye that of snakes.

Bezzubova tells the story of another extreme relationship with the smart-phone. Shy but thirsty for attention, Cornelia composed a long list of things about herself that she was ashamed of and wanted to change, from the color of her hair to the tone of her voice. She hated herself and her life. For her 12th birthday her parents presented her with her first smartphone. She discovered her own new digital world with its social platforms, messenger services, on-line games, and other possibilities for her virtual presence and communica-tion. "Building my profiles on social media became my second birth! I was not ashamed of myself anymore. I created a new self and I was proud of it," she reportedly said. Fascinated by their daughter's enthusiasm, her parents supported her absorption in digital life. The realization of the rift between her virtual life and real life came along with the shocking and tragic news that Cornelia was terminally ill. The family provided love and support. But Cornelia believed that her virtual self was the truest expression of who she was (p. 100).[5]

Inspired by the gravestone of a 25-year-old woman in Russia, she asked that her own memorial be in the shape of an iPhone emblazoned with her fa-vorite selfie. She wanted to be remembered this way, so her wish was honored. The smartphone in some way provided the sense of security necessary for her to build elements of an independent life, though limited by cyberspace—a virtual independent life. Her relationship with the smartphone had features of the relationships with a self-object—that is, a narcissistically imbued virtual self. Her choice to be remembered as her virtual self represents the dramatic impact that the mixture of the real and the virtual can potentially make on a young person's life.

"In a broad cultural context a gravestone might be seen as the ultimate image of self, the final mask," Bezzubova observes (p. 100).[5] The one in the shape of a smartphone with a selfie symbolizes the presence of the virtual self in contemporary life. While these instances are extreme, there is little doubt that technology will continue at its meteoric pace, unhindered by negative impacts on individual selves.

"As we distribute ourselves, we may abandon ourselves," warns Turkle (p. 12).[1] Will machines make us less human? Or will technology bring us closer to answering Gauguin's existential questions? With every change there will be criticism and debate. And if the line defining what's real and what is not continues to blur unchecked, the fault may lie not in our stars, but in ourselves and our technology.

References

Chapter 1

1. Styron, W. (1990). *Darkness visible*. Vintage Books. Quotes are on pp. 7, 38.
2. Dugas, L. (1898). Un cas de dépersonalisation. *Revue Philosophique, 55*, 500–507.
3. Amiel, H. F. (1882/1906). *The journal intime of Henri-Frédéric Amiel* (H. Ward, trans.). Macmillan. Quote is on pp. 304–305.
4. Freud, S. (1936). A disturbance of memory on the Acropolis. In *Standard Edition of Complete Works of Sigmund Freud* (vol. 22). Hogarth Press.
5. Noyes, A. P., & Kolb, L. (1939/1964). *Modern clinical psychiatry* (6th ed.). W. B. Saunders. Quote is on p. 84.
6. American Psychiatric Association. (2022). *Diagnostic and statistical manual of mental disorders* (5th ed., text rev.).
7. Myers, D. (1972). A study of depersonalization in students. *British Journal of Psychiatry, 121*, 62.
8. Noyes, R., Hoenk, P. R., Kuperman, S., & Slymen, D. J. (1977). Depersonalization in accident victims and psychiatric patients. *Journal of Nervous and Mental Disorders, 164*(6), 401–407.
9. Hunter, E. C., Sierra, M., & David, A. S. (2004). The epidemiology of depersonalisation and derealization: A systematic review. *Social Psychiatry and Psychiatric Epidemiology, 38*(1), 9–18.

Chapter 2

1. Schilder, P. (1939). The treatment of depersonalization. *The Bulletin, Psychiatric Division of Bellevue Hospital*, p. 260.
2. Zeller, A. (1838). Uber einige Hauptpunkte in der Erforschung und Heilung der *Seelenstorungen. Zeitschrift fur die Beurtheilung und heilung der krankhafte Seelenzustande, 1*, 515–559. As cited in Sierra, M. (2009). *Depersonalization: A New Look at a Neglected Syndrome*. Cambridge: Cambridge University Press, p. 8.
3. Esquirol, J. E. (1838). *Des maladies mentales* (vol. I). Bailliere.
4. Billod, E. (1847). Maladies de la volante. *Annales Medico-Psychologiques, 10*, 15–35; 170–202; 317–47. As cited in Sierra, M. (2009). *Depersonalization: A New Look at a Neglected Syndrome*. Cambridge: Cambridge University Press, p. 8.
5. Griesinger, W. (1845). Ueber einige epileptoide Zustande. *Archiv fur Psychiatrie und Nervenkrankheiten, I*, 320–333. As cited in Sierra, M. (2009). *Depersonalization: A New Look at a Neglected Syndrome*. Cambridge: Cambridge University Press, p. 8.
6. Krishaber, M. (1873). *De la neuropathie cerebro-cardiaque*. G. Masson, p. 10.
7. Dugas, L. (1898). Un case de dépersonalisation. *Revue Philosophique, 45*, 500–506.

8. Phillips, M. L., Medford, N., Senior, C., Bullmore, E., Suckling, J., Brammer, M., Andrew, C., Sierra, M., Williams, S. C., & David, A. S. (2001). Depersonalization disorder: Thinking without feeling. *Psychiatry Research: Neuroimaging, 108*, 145–160.

9 . Ribot, T. (1895). *Les maladies de la personnalite* (6th ed.). Felix Alcan. As cited in Sierra, M. (2009). *Depersonalization: A New Look at a Neglected Syndrome.* Cambridge: Cambridge University Press, p. 8.

10. Wernicke, C. (1906). *Drundriss der Psychiatrie in Klinischen Vorlesungen* (2nd ed.). Georg Thieme. As cited in Sierra, M. (2009). *Depersonalization: A New Look at a Neglected Syndrome.* Cambridge: Cambridge University Press, p. 11.

11. Pick, A. (1909). Zur Pathologie des Ich Bewusstweins. *Archiv fur Psychiatrie un Nervenkrankheiten, 38*, 22–23.

12. Foerster, O. (1903). Ein Fall von elementarer allgemeiner Somatopsychose (Afunction der Somatopsyche). *Monatsschrift fur Psychiatrie und Neurologie, 14*, 189–205. As cited in Sierra, M. (2009). *Depersonalization: A New Look at a Neglected Syndrome.* Cambridge: Cambridge University Press, p. 11.

13 . Janet, P. (1903). *Les obsessions et la psychasthenie.* Alcan, p. 106.

14. Amiel, H. F. (1882/1906). *The journal intime of Henri-Frédéric Amiel* (H. Ward, trans.). Macmillan, pp. 304–305.

15. Kraepelin, E. (1887). Uber Erinnerungsfalschungen. *Archiv fur Psychiatrie und Nervenkrankheiten, 18*, 395–436. As cited in Sierra, M. (2009). *Depersonalization: A New Look at a Neglected Syndrome.* Cambridge: Cambridge University Press, p. 12.

16. Shafer, O. (1880). Bemerkungen zur psychiatrischen Formenlehre. *Allgemeine Zeitschrift fur Psychiatrie, 36*, 214–278. As cited in Sierra, M. (2009). *Depersonalization: A New Look at a Neglected Syndrome.* Cambridge: Cambridge University Press, p. 13.

17. Storring, G. (1900). *Vorlesungen uber Psychopathologie in threr Bedeutung fur de normale Psychologie.* Kessinger Publishing. As cited in Sierra, M. (2009). *Depersonalization: A New Look at a Neglected Syndrome.* Cambridge: Cambridge University Press, p. 13.

18. Lowy, M. (1908). Die Aktionsgefuhle: Ein Depeersonalisationfall als Betrag Zur Psychologie des Aktivitatsgefuhles und des Personlichkeitbewusstseins. *Prager Medizinische Wochenschrift, 33*, 443–461. As cited in Sierra, M. (2009). *Depersonalization: A New Look at a Neglected Syndrome.* Cambridge: Cambridge University Press, p. 14.

19 . Janet, P. (1928). *De l'angoisses a la extase.* Alcan.

20. Mayer-Gross, W. (1935). On depersonalization. *British Journal of Medicine and Psychology, 15*, 103–126.

21. James, W. (1902/1961). *The varieties of religious experience.* Macmillan. Quote is on p. 66.

22 . Freud, S. (1936/1964). *A Disturbance of Memory on the Acropolis, Standard Edition* 22: 237–248. Quotes are from Vol. 22, pp. 239–248.

23. Freud, S. (1936/1964). *From the History of an Infantile Neurosis, Standard Edition* 17: 7–122.

24. Freud, S. (Ed.). (1971–1919). The "Uncanny." In *The Standard Edition of the Complete Psychological Works of Sigmund Freud*, Vol. XVII: *An Infantile Neurosis and Other Works*: 217–256.

25. Federn, P. (1953). *Ego psychology and the psychoses.* Imago Publishing.

26. Oberndorf, C. P. (1934). Depersonalization in relation to erotization of thought. *International Journal of Psychoanalysis, 15*, 271–295.

27. Oberndorf, C. P. (1950). The role of anxiety in depersonalisation. *International Journal of Psychoanalysis, 31*, 1–5.
28. Schilder, P. (1953). *Medical psychology*. International Universities Press, pp. 305–306, 310.
29. Wittels, F. (1940). Psychology and treatment of depersonalization. *Psychoanalytic Review, 27*, 57.
30. Jacobson, E. (1959). Depersonalization. *Journal of the American Psychoanalytic Association, 7*, 581.
31. Sarlin, C. N. (1962). Depersonalization and derealization. *Journal of the American Psychoanalytic Association, 10*, 784.
32. Arlow, J. A. (1966). Depersonalization and derealization. In R. M. Loewenstein, L. M. Newman, M. Schur, & A. J. Solnit (Eds.), *Psychoanalysis: A general psychology* (pp. 456–477). International Universities Press.
33. Jaspers, K. (1948). *Allgemeine Psychopathologie* (5th ed.). Springer.
34. Shorvon, H. J. (1946). The depersonalization syndrome. *Proceedings of the Royal Society of Medicine, 34*, 779–792.
35. Roth, M. R. (1960). The phobic anxiety-depersonalization syndrome and some general aetiological problems in psychiatry. *Journal of Neuropsychiatry, 1*, 293–306.
36. Roth, M., & Argyle, N. (1988). Anxiety panic and phobic disorder: An overview. *Journal of Psychiatric Research, 22*(supp 1), 33–54.
37. Torch, E. M. (1978). Review of the relation between obsession/depersonalization. *Acta Psychiatrica Scandinavica, 58*, 191–198. Quote is on p. 194.
38. Noyes, R., Jr., Kletti, R., & Kupperman, X. (1977). Depersonalization in response to life threatening danger. *Comprehensive Psychiatry, 18*, 375–384.
39. James, W. (1892). The Self. As cited in J. Pooley (Ed.), *Social Media & the Self: An Open Reader* (1st ed.). mediastudies.press. https://doi.org/10.32376/3f8575cb.8ccffaec.
40. Cattell, J. P., & Cattell, J. S. (1974). Depersonalization: Psychological and social perspectives. In Silvano Arieti (Ed.), *American handbook of psychiatry* (pp. 766–799). Basic Books, p. 768.
41. Bettelheim, B. (1967). *The empty fortress*. Free Press. Quoted in Cattell & Cattell, p. 773.
42. Laing, R. D. (1965). *The divided self*. Penguin Books. As cited in Gordon, James S. (1990). Understanding the secret self. *The Washington Post*, June 12. https://www.washingtonpost.com/archive/lifestyle/wellness/1990/06/12/understanding-the-secret-self/1ef214e0-eadb-4b5f-89c6-634a9f759cb9/.

Chapter 3

1. Radovic, F., & Radovic, S. (2002). Feelings of unreality: A conceptual and phenomenological analysis of the language of depersonalization. *Philosophy, Psychiatry, and Psychology, 9*(3), 271–279.
2. Bernstein-Carlson, E., & Putnam, F. W. (1993). An update on the Dissociative Experiences Scale. *Dissociation, 6*, 16–27.
3. Simeon, D., Guralnik, O., Gross, S., Stein, D. J., Schmeidler, J., & Hollander, E. (1998). The detection and measurement of depersonalization disorder. *Journal of Nervous and Mental Disease, 186*, 536–542.
4. Sierra, M., & Berrios, G. E. (2001). The phenomenological stability of depersonalization: Comparing the old with the new. *Journal of Nervous and Mental Disease, 189*(9), 629–636.

5. Sierra, M., & Berrios, G. E. (2000). The Cambridge Depersonalization Scale: A new instrument for the measurement of depersonalization. *Psychiatry Research, 93*, 153–164.
6. Michal, M., Glaesmer, H., Zwerentz, R., Knebel, A., Wiltink, J., Brahler, E., & Beutel, M. E. (2010). Base rates for depersonalization according to the 2-item version of the Cambridge Depersonalization Scale (CDS-2) and its associations with depression/anxiety in the general population. *Journal of Affective Disorders, 128*, 106–111.
7. Simeon, D., Kozin, D. S., Segal, K., Lerch, B., Dujour, R., & Giesbrecht, T. (2008). Deconstructing depersonalization: Further evidence for symptom clusters. *Psychiatry Research, 157*, 303–306.

Chapter 4

1. American Psychiatric Association. (2022). *Diagnostic and statistical manual of mental disorders* (5th ed., text rev.).
2. American Psychiatric Association. (1980). *Diagnostic and statistical manual of mental disorders* (3rd ed.).
3. Bernstein-Carlson, E., & Putnam, F. W. (1993). An update on the Dissociative Experiences Scale. *Dissociation, 6*, 16–27.
4. Sierra, M., & Berrios, G. E. (2000). The Cambridge Depersonalisation Scale: A new instrument for the measurement of depersonalization. *Psychiatry Research, 93*, 153–164.

Chapter 5

1. American Psychiatric Association. (2022). *Diagnostic and statistical manual of mental disorders* (5th ed., text rev.).
2. Bernstein-Carlson, E., & Putnam, F. W. (1993). An update on the Dissociative Experiences Scale. *Dissociation, 6*, 16–27.
3. Simeon, D., Knutelska, M., Nelson, D., & Guralnik, O. (2003). Feeling unreal: A depersonalization disorder update of 117 cases. *Journal of Clinical Psychiatry, 64*, 990–997.
4. Kumar, A., & Cohen, C. (2021). Panic disorder in older adults: Two case reports. *American Journal of Geriatric Psychiatry, 29*(4), S58–S59.
5. Lambert, M. V., Sierra, M., Phillips, M., & David, A. S. (2002). The spectrum of organic depersonalization: A review plus four new cases. *Journal of Neuropsychiatry, 14*, 141–154.

Chapter 6

1. Simeon, D., & Putnam, F. (2022). Pathological dissociation in the National Comorbidity Survey Replication (NCS-R): Prevalence, morbidity, comorbidity, and childhood maltreatment. *Journal of Trauma and Dissociation, 23*(5), 490–503 (online ahead of print). doi:10.1080/15299732.2022.2064580
2. Aderibigbe, Y. A., Bloch, R. M., & Walker, W. R. (2001). Prevalence of depersonalization and derealization experiences in a rural population. *Social Psychiatry and Psychiatric Epidemiology, 36*, 63–69.

3. Hunter, E. C., Sierra, M., & David, A. S. (2004). The epidemiology of realization ion and derealization: A systematic review. *Social Psychiatry and Psychiatric Epidemiology, 39*, 9–18.

4. Michal, M., Wiltnik, J., Subic-Wrana, C., Zwerenz, R., Tuin, I., Lichy, M., Brähler, E., & Beutel, M. E. (2009). Prevalence, correlates, and predictors of depersonalization experiences in the German general population. *Journal of Nervous and Mental Disease, 197*(7), 499–506.

5. Ross, C. (1991). The epidemiology of multiple personality disorder and dissociation. *Psychiatric Clinics of North America, 14*, 503–517.

6. Johnson, J. G., Cohen, P., Kasen, S., & Brook, J.S. (2006). Dissociative disorders among adults in the community, impaired functioning, and axis I and II comorbidity. *Journal of Psychiatric Research, 40*, 131–140.

7. Sar, V., Akyüz, G., & Doğan, O. (2007). Prevalence of dissociative disorders among women in the general population. *Psychiatry Research, 149*, 169–176.

8. Simeon, D., Knutelska, M., Nelson, D., & Guralnik, O. (2003). Feeling unreal: A depersonalization disorder update of 117 cases. *Journal of Clinical Psychiatry, 64*, 990–997.

9. Baker, D., Hunter, E., Lawrence, E., Medford, N., Patel, M., Senior, C., Sierra, M., Lambert, M. V., Phillips, M. L., & David, A. S. (2003). Depersonalisation disorder: Clinical features of 204 cases. *British Journal of Psychiatry, 182*, 428–433·

10. Michal, M., Adler, J., Wiltink, J., Reiner, I., Tschan, R., Wolfling, K., Weimert, S., Tuiin, I., Subic-Wrana, C., Beutel, M. E., & Zwerenz, R. (2016). A case series of 223 patients with depersonalization-derealization syndrome. *BMC Psychiatry, 16*, 203–213.

11. Lanius, R. A., Vermetten, E., Loewenstein, R. J., Brand, B., Schmahl, C., Bremner, J. D., & Spiegel, D. (2010). Emotion modulation in PTSD: Clinical and neurobiological evidence for a dissociative subtype. *American Journal of Psychiatry, 167*(6), 640–647.

12. Waller, N. G., & Ross, C. A. (1997). The prevalence and biometric structure of pathological dissociation in the general population: Taxometric and behavior genetic findings. *Journal of Abnormal Psychology, 106*, 499–510.

13. Jang, K. L., Paris, J., Zweig-Frank, H., & Livesley, W. J. (1998). Twin study of dissociative experience. *Journal of Nervous and Mental Disease, 186*, 345–351.

14. Becker-Blease, K. A., Deater-Deckard, K., Eley, T., Freyd, J. J., Stevenson, J., & Plomin, R. (2004). A genetic analysis of individual differences in dissociative behaviors in childhood and adolescence. *Journal of Child Psychology and Psychiatry, 45*(3), 522–532.

15. Putnam, F. W. (2016). *The way we are: How states of mind influence our identities, personality and potential for change*. Ipbooks.

16. Szymanski, H. V. (1981). Prolonged depersonalization after marijuana use. *American Journal of Psychiatry, 138*, 231–233.

17. Keshaven, M. S., & Lishman W. A. (1986). Prolonged depersonalization following cannabis abuse. *British Journal of Addiction, 81*, 140–142.

18. Medford, N., Baker, D., Hunter, E., Sierra, M., Lawrence, E., Phillips, M. L., & David, A. S. (2003). Chronic depersonalization following illicit drug use: A controlled analysis of 40 cases. *Addiction, 98*, 1711–1716.

19. Simeon, D., Kozin, D. S., Segal, K., & Lerch, B. (2009). Is depersonalization disorder initiated by illicit drug use any different? A survey of 394 adults. *Journal of Clinical Psychiatry, 70*(10), 1358–1364.

20. National Institute of Drug Abuse. (2021, April 13). How does marijuana produce its effects? https://nida.nih.gov/publications/research-reports/marijuana/how-does-marijuana-produce-its-effects.

21. Ramikie, T. S., Nyilas, R., Bluett, R. J., Gamble-George, J. C., Hartley, N. D., Mackie, K., Watanabe, M., Katona, I., & Patel, S. (2014). Multiple mechanistically distinct modes of endocannabinoid mobilization at central amygdala glutamatergic synapses. *Neuron, 81*(5), 1111–1125.

22. Vignault, C., Masse, A., Gouron, D., Quintin, J., Asli, K. D., & Semaan, W. (2021). The potential impact of recreational cannabis legalization on the prevalence of cannabis use disorder and psychotic disorders: A retrospective observational study. *Canadian Journal of Psychiatry, 66*(12), 1069–1076.

23. Gouron, D., Vignault, C., Quintin, J., Semaan, W., & Asli, K. D. (2020). Impacts de la legalization du cannabis recreative sure la sante mentale: Une recension des ecrits. *Sante Mentale au Quebec, 45*(1), 201–220.

24. Sarris, J., Sinclair, J., Karamacoska, D., Davidson, M., & Firth, J. (2020). Medicinal cannabis for psychiatric disorders: A clinically-focused systematic review. *BMC Psychiatry, 20*, article 24.

Chapter 7

1. Felitti, V. J., Anda, R. F., Nordenberg, D., Williamson, D. F., Spitz, A. M., Edwards, V., Koss, M. P., & Marks, J. S. (1998). Relationship of childhood abuse and household dysfunction to many of the leading causes of death in adults: The Adverse Childhood Experiences (ACE) study. *American Journal of Preventive Medicine, 14*, 245–258.

2. American Psychiatric Association. (2022). *Diagnostic and statistical manual of mental disorders* (5th ed., text rev.).

3. Simeon, D., & Putnam, F. (2022). Pathological dissociation in the National Comorbidity Survey Replication (NCS-R): Prevalence, morbidity, comorbidity, and childhood maltreatment. *Journal of Trauma & Dissociation, 23*(5), 490–503 (online ahead of print). doi:10.1080/15299732.2022.2064580

4. Simeon, D., Guralnik, O., Schmeidler, J., Sirof, B., & Knutelska, M. (2001). The role of childhood interpersonal trauma in depersonalization disorder. *American Journal of Psychiatry, 158*, 1027–1033.

5. Bernstein, D. P., Stein, J. A., Newcomb, M. D., Walkter, E., Pogge, D., Ahluvalia T, Stokes, J., Handelsman, L., Medrano, M., Desmond, D., & Zule, W. (2003). Development and validation of a brief screening version of the Childhood Trauma Questionnaire. *Child Abuse & Neglect, 27*, 169–190.

6. Simeon, D., Knutelska, M., Yehuda, R., Putnam, F., Schmeidler, J., & Smith, L. M. (2007). Hypothalamic-pituitary-adrenal axis function in dissociative disorders, post-traumatic stress disorder, and healthy volunteers. *Biological Psychiatry, 61*, 966–973.

7. Walker E. A., Unutzer, J., Rutter, C., Gelfand, A., Saunders, K., VonKorff, M., Koss, M. P., & Katon, W. (1999 July). Costs of health care use by women HMO members with a history of childhood abuse and neglect. *Archives of General Psychiatry, 56*(7), 609–613. doi: 10.1001/archpsyc.56.7.609. PMID: 10401506.

8. Personal communication, Simeon, D.

9. Lemche, E., Brammer, M. J., David, A. S., Surguladze, S. A., Phillips, M. L., Sierra, M., Williams, S. C. R., & Giampietro, V. P. (2013). Interoceptive-reflective regions differentiate alexithyma traits in depersonalization disorder. *Psychiatry Research: Neuroimaging, 214*, 66–72.

10. Michal, M., Adler, J., Wiltink, J., Reiner, I., Tschan, R., Wolfling, K., Weimert, S., Tuiin, I., Subic-Wrana, C., Beutel, M. E., & Zwerenz, R. (2016). A case series of 223 patients with depersonalization-derealization syndrome. *BMC Psychiatry, 16*, 203–213.

11. Lippard, E. T. C., & Nemeroff, C. B. (2020). The devastating clinical consequences of child abuse and neglect: Increased disease vulnerability and poor treatment response in mood disorders. *American Journal of Psychiatry, 177*(1), 20–36.

12. Michal, M., Wiltnik, J., Subic-Wrana, C., Zwerenz, R., Tuin, I., Lichy, M., Brähler, E., & Beutel, M. E. (2009). Prevalence, correlates, and predictors of depersonalization experiences in the German general population. *Journal of Nervous and Mental Disease, 197*(7), 499–506.

13. Thomson, P., & Jaque, S. V. (2018). Depersonalization, adversity, emotionality, and coping with stressful situations. *Journal of Trauma and Dissociation, 19*(2), 143–161.

14. Laoide, A. O., Egan, J., & Osborn, K. (2018). What was once essential, may become detrimental: The mediating role of depersonalization in the relationship between childhood emotional maltreatment and psychological distress in adults. *Journal of Trauma & Dissociation, 19*, 514–534.

15. Someon, D. Personal communication.

16. Hesse, E., & Main, M. (1999). Second-generation effects of unresolved trauma in nonmaltreating parents: Dissociated, frightened, and threatening parental behavior. *Psychoanalytic Inquiry, 19*(4):481–540.

17. Coe, M. T., Dalenberg, C. J., Aransky, K. M., & Reto, C. S. (1995). Adult attachment style, reported childhood violence history and types of dissociative experiences. *Dissociation, 8*, 142–154.

18. Simeon, D., & Knutelska, M. (2022). The role of fearful attachment in depersonalization disorder. *European Journal of Trauma & Dissociation, 6*(3a), 100266.

19. Young, J., Klosko, J. S., & Weishaar, M. E. (2003). *Schema therapy: A practitioner's guide* (1st ed.). Guilford Press.

20. Simeon, D., Guralnik, O., Knutelska, M., & Schmeidler, J. (2002). Personality factors associated with dissociation: Temperament, defenses and cognitive schemata. *American Journal of Psychiatry, 159*, 489–491.

21. Tang, A., Crawford, H., Morales, S., Degnan, K. A., Pine, D. S., & Fox, N. (2020). Infant behavioral inhibition predicts personality and social outcomes three decades later. *Proceedings of the National Academy of Sciences, 117*(18), 9800–9807.

22. Bagby, R. M., Parker, J. D. A, & Taylor, G. J. (1993). The twenty-item Toronto Alexithymia Scale—I. Item selection and cross-validation of the factor structure. *Journal of Psychosomatic Research, 38*(1), 23–32.

23. Simeon, D., Giesbrecht, T., Knutelska, M., Smith, R. J., & Smith, L. M. (2009). Alexithymia, absorption, and cognitive failures in depersonalization disorder: A comparison to posttraumatic stress disorder and healthy volunteers. *Journal of Nervous and Mental Disease, 197*, 492–498.

24. Lemche, E., Brammer, M. J., David, A. S., Surguladze, S. A., Phillips, M. L., Sierra, M., Williams, S. C. R., & Giampietro, V. P. (2013). Interoceptive-reflective regions differentiate alexithyma traits in depersonalization disorder. *Psychiatry Research: Neuroimaging, 214*, 66–72.

25. Michal, M., Beutel, M. E., Jordan, J., Zimmermann, M., Wolters, S., & Heidenreich, T. (2007). Depersonalization, mindfulness, and childhood trauma. *Journal of Nervous and Mental Disease, 195*, 693–696.

26. Guralnik, O., Schmeidler, J., & Simeon, D. (2000). Feeling unreal: Cognitive processes in depersonalization. *American Journal of Psychiatry, 157*, 103–109.

27. Guralnik, O., Giesbrecht, T., Knutelska, M., Sirroff, B., & Simeon, D. (2007). Cognitive functioning in depersonalization disorder. *Journal of Nervous and Mental Disease, 195,* 983–988.

28. Simeon, D., Knutelska, M., Putnam, F. W., Schmeidler, J., & Smith, L. M. (2022). Attention and memory in depersonalization-spectrum dissociative disorders: impact of selective-divided attentional condition, stimulus emotionality, and stress. *Journal of Trauma and Dissociation* May 26, 1–21. doi:10.1080/15299732.2022.2079798c

Chapter 8

1. Vallar, G., & Perani, D. (1986). The anatomy of unilateral neglect after right-hemisphere stroke lesions: A clinical/CT-scan correlation study in man. *Neuropsychologia, 24*(5), 609–622.

2. Ackner, B. (1954). Depersonalization: I. Aetiology and phenomenology. *Journal of Mental Science, 100*(421), 838–853.

3. Salanova, V., Andermann, F., Rasmussen, T., Olivier, A., & Quesney, L. F. (1995). Parietal lobe epilepsy: Clinical manifestations and outcome in 82 patients treated surgically between 1929 and 1988. *Brain, 118*(3), 607–627.

4. Blanke, O., Ortigue, S., Landis, T., & Seeck, M. (2002). Stimulating illusory own-body perceptions. *Nature, 419*(6904), 269–270.

5. Penfield, W., & Rasmussen, T. (1950). *The cerebral cortex of man: A clinical study of localization of function.* Macmillan.

6. Devinsky, O., Putnam, F., Grafman, J., Bromfield, E., & Theodore, W. H. (1989). Dissociative states and epilepsy. *Neurology, 39*(6), 835–840.

7. Gorno-Tempini, M. L., Price, C. J., Josephs, O., Vandenberghe, R., Cappa, S. F., Kapur, N., & Frackowiak, R. S. (1998). The neural systems sustaining face and proper-name processing. *Brain, 121*(11), 2103–2118.

8. Simeon, D., Guralnik, O., Hazlett, E. A., Spiegel-Cohen, J., Hollander, E., & Buchsbaum, M. S. (2000). Feeling unreal: A PET study of depersonalization disorder. *American Journal of Psychiatry, 157,* 1782–1788.

9. Adolphs, R., Damasio, H., Tranel, D., Cooper, G., & Damasio, A. R. (2000). A role for somatosensory cortices in the visual recognition of emotion as revealed by three-dimensional lesion mapping. *Journal of Neuroscience, 20*(7), 2683–2690.

10. Blanke, O., Mohr, C., Michel, C. M., Pascual-Leone, A., Brugger, P., Seeck, M., Landis, T., & Thut, G. (2005). Linking out-of-body experience and self processing to mental own-body imagery at the temporoparietal junction. *Journal of Neuroscience, 25*(3), 550–557.

11. Krystal, J. H., Bremner, D. J., Southwick, S. M., & Charney, D. S. (1998). The emerging neurobiology of dissociation: Implications for the treatment of posttraumatic stress disorder. In D. J. Bremner and C. R. Marmar (Eds.), *Trauma, Memory and Dissociation* (pp. 321–358). Washington, DC: American Psychiatric Press, Inc.

12. Hughes, K. C., & Shin, L. M. (2011). Functional neuroimaging studies of post-traumatic stress disorder. *Expert Review of Neurotherapeutics, 11*(2), 275–285.

13. LeDoux, J. (1996). *The emotional brain.* Simon & Schuster.

14. Gogolia, N. (2017). The insular cortex. *Current Biology, 27,* R573–R591.

15. Sierra, M., & Berrios, G. E. (1998). Depersonalization: Neurobiological perspectives. *Biological Psychiatry, 44*(9), 898–908.

16. Matthew, R. J., Wilson, W. H., Chiu, N. Y., Turkington, T. G., Degrado, T. R., & Coleman, R. E. (1999). Regional cerebral blood flow and depersonalization after tetrahydrocannabinol administration. *Acta Psychiatrica Scandinavica, 100*(1), 67–75.

17. Phillips, M. L., Medford, N., Senior, C., Bullmore, E., Suckling, J., Brammer, M., Andrew, C., Sierra, M., Williams, S. C., & David, A. S. (2001). Depersonalization disorder: Thinking without feeling. *Psychiatry Research: Neuroimaging, 108*, 145–160.

18. Ekman, P. (1992). An argument for basic emotions. *Cognition and Emotion, 6*, 169–200.

19. Lemche, E., Anikumar, A., Giampetro, V. P., Brammer, M. J., Surgulaze, S. A., Lawrence, N. S., Gasston, D., Chitnis, X., Williams, S. C. R., Sierra, M., Joraschky, P., & Phillips, M. L. (2008). Cerebral and autonomic responses to emotional facial expressions in depersonalization disorder. *British Journal of Psychiatry, 193*, 222–228.

20. Medford, N., Sierra, M., Stringaris, A., Giampietro, V., Bremmer, M. J., & David, A. S. (2016). Emotional experience and awareness of self: Functional MRI studies of depersonalization disorder. *Frontiers in Psychology, 7*, article 432.

21. Medford, N., Brierley, B., Brammer, M., Bullmore, E. T., David, A. S., & Phillips, M. L. (2006). Emotional memory in depersonalization disorder: A functional MRI study. *Psychiatry Research: Neuroimaging, 148*(2–3), 93–102.

22. Lemche, E., Brammer, M. J., David, A. S., Surguladze, S. A., Phillips, M. A., Sierra, M., Williams, S. C. R., & Giampietro, V. P. (2013). Interoceptive-reflective regions differentiate alexithymia traits in depersonalization disorder. *Psychiatry Research: Neuroimaging, 214*, 66–72.

23. Lanius, R. A., Brand, B., Vermetten, E., Frewen, P. A., & Spiegel, D. (2012). The dissociative subtype of posttraumatic stress disorder: Rationale, clinical and neurobiological evidence, and implications. *Depression and Anxiety, 29*, 701–8. doi: 10.1002/Da.21889.

24. Griffin, M. G., Resick, P. A., & Mechanic, M. B. (1997). Objective assessment of peritraumatic dissociation: Psychophysiological indicators. *American Journal of Psychiatry, 154*(8), 1081–1088.

25. Sierra, M., Senior, C., Dalton, J., McDonough, M., Bond, A., Phillips, M. L., O'Dwyer, A. M., & David, A. S. (2002). Autonomic response in depersonalization disorder. *Archives of General Psychiatry, 59*, 833–838.

26. Sierra, M., Senior, C., Phillips, M. L., & David, A. S. (2006). Autonomic response in the perception of disgust and happiness in depersonalization disorder. *Psychiatry Research, 145*(2–3), 225–231.

27. Michal, M., Koechel, A., Canterino, M., Adler, J., Reiner, I., Vossel, G., Beutel, M. E., & Gamer, M. (2013). Depersonalization disorder: Disconnection of cognitive evaluation from autonomic responses to emotional stimuli. *PLoS ONE, 8*(9), e74331.

28. Simeon, D., Guralnik, O., Knutelska, M., Yehuda, R., & Schmeidler, J. (2003). Basal norepinephrine in depersonalization disorder. *Psychiatry Research, 121*, 93–97.

29. Simeon, D., Knutelska, M., Smith, L., Baker, B. R., & Hollander, E. (2007). A preliminary study of cortisol and norepinephrine reactivity to psychosocial stress in borderline personality disorder with high and low dissociation. *Psychiatry Research, 149*, 177–184.

30. Delahanty, D., Royer, D., Raimonde, A. J., & Spoonster, E. (2003). Peritraumatic dissociation is inversely related to catecholamine levels in initial urine samples of motor vehicle accident victims. *Journal of Trauma & Dissociation, 4*(1), 65–80.

31. Owens, A. P., David, A. S., Low, D. A., Mathias, C. J., & Sierra-Siegert, M. (2015). Abnormal cardiovascular sympathetic and parasympathetic responses to physical and emotional stimuli in depersonalization disorder. *Frontiers in Neuroscience, 9,* article 89.

32. Simeon, D., Guralnik, O., Knutelska, M., Hollander, E., & Schmeidler, J. (2001). Hypothalamic-pituitary-adrenal axis dysregulation in depersonalization disorder. *Neuropsychopharmacology, 25,* 793–795.

33. Simeon, D., Knutelska, M., Yehuda, R., Putnam, F., Schmeidler, J., & Smith, L. M. (2007). Hypothalamic-pituitary-adrenal axis function in dissociative disorders, post-traumatic stress disorder, and healthy volunteers. *Biological Psychiatry, 61,* 966–973.

34. Simeon, D., Knutelska, M., Nelson, D., & Guralnik, O. (2003). Feeling unreal: A depersonalization disorder update of 117 cases. *Journal of Clinical Psychiatry, 64,* 990–997.

35. Simeon, D., Hollander, E., Saoud, J. B., DeCaria, C., Cohen, L., Stein, D. J., Islam, M. N., & Hwang, M. (1995). Induction of depersonalization by the serotonin agonist m-CPP. *Psychiatry Research, 58,* 161–164.

36. Southwick, S., Krystal, J., Bremner, D., Morgan, C. A., Nicolaou, A., Johnson, D., Heninger, G., & Charney, D. (1997). Noradrenergic and serotonergic function in posttraumatic stress disorder. *Archives of General Psychiatry, 54*(8), 749–758.

37. Pitman, R. K., van der Kolk, B. A., Orr, S. P., & Greenberg, M. S. (1990). Naloxone-reversible analgesic response to combat-related stimuli in posttraumatic stress disorder. *Archives of General Psychiatry, 47*(6), 541–544.

38. Walsh, S. L., Geter-Douglas, B., Strain, E. C., & Bigelow, G. E. (2001). Enadoline and butorphanol: Evaluation of kappa-agonists on cocaine pharmacodynamics and cocaine self-administration in humans. *Journal of Pharmacology & Experimental Therapeutics, 299*(1), 147–158.

39. Daniels, J. K., Gaebler, M., Lamke J-P., & Walter, H. (2015). Grey matter alterations in patients with depersonalization disorder: A voxel-based morphometry study. *Journal of Psychiatry & Neuroscience, 40*(1), 19–27.

40. Vesuna, S., Kauvar, I. V., Richman, E., Gore, F., Oskotsky, T., Sava-Segal, C., Luo, L., Malenka, R. C., Henderson, J. M., Nuyujukian, P., Parvizi, J., & Deisseroth, K. (2020). Deep posteromedial cortical rhythm in dissociation. *Nature, 586*(7827), 87–94.

41. Ketay, S., Hamilton, H. K., Haas, B. W., & Simeon, D. (2014). Face processing in depersonalization: An fMRI study of the unfamiliar self. *Psychiatry Research, 222*(1–2), 107–110.

Chapter 9

1. Pascal, B. (1995). *Pensées.* Penguin Books, p. 19.

2. Amiel, H. F. (1885/1906). *The journal intime of Henri-Frédéric Amiel* (H. Ward, trans.). Macmillan.

3. Nemiah, J. C. (1989). Depersonalization disorder (depersonalization neurosis). In H. I. Kaplan & B. J. Sadock (Eds.), *Comprehensive textbook of psychiatry* (5th ed., vol. 1, pp. 1038–1044). Williams & Wilkins, p. 1042.

4. Woolf, V. (1985). *Moments of being: A collection of autobiographical writing.* Harvest Books.

5. Sartre, J. P. (1938/1962). *Nausea.* New Directions Publishing Corp.

6. Nieli, R. (1987). *Wittgenstein: From mystery to ordinary language.* SUNY Press, p. 30.
7. Camus, A. (1942/1946). *The stranger.* Vintage Books.
8. Dugas, L. (1898). Un cas de dépersonalisation. *Revue Philosophique, 45,* 500–507.
9. de Caussade, J.-P. (1731). Excerpt from a letter to sister Mary-Antoinette de Mahuet.
10. Roberts, B. (1993). *The experience of no-self.* SUNY Press.
11. Roberts, B. (1991). *The path to no-self: Life at the center.* Alabany: State University of New York Press, p. 27.
12. Segal, S. (1996/1998). *Collision with the infinite.* Blue Dove Press.
13. Huxley, A. (1963). *The doors of perception: and heaven and hell.* Harper and Row.
14. Janiger, O., & Dobkin de Rios, M. (2003). *LSD, spirituality and the creative process.* Park Street Press.
15. Wilson, C. (1956/1978). *The outsider.* Pan Books Ltd.
16. Newberg, A. Questions and answers online interview. https://psyche.co/ideas/how-an-intense-spiritual-retreat-might-change-your-brain
17. Newberg, A. (2022). *How an intense spiritual retreat might change your brain.* Psyche, Aeon Newsletter. https://psyche.co/ideas/how-an-intense-spiritual-retreat-might-change-your-brain
18.. Mphanza, C. (2022). *Frame Six, The Rinehard Frames.* Lincoln: University of Nebraska Press.

Chapter 10

1. Schilder, P. (1939). The treatment of depersonalization. *Bulletin of the New York Academy of Medicine, 15,* 258–272.
2. Davison, K. (1964). Episodic depersonalization: Observations on 7 patients. *British Journal of Psychiatry, 110,* 505–513.
3. King, A., & Little, J. (1959). Thiopentone treatment of the phobic anxiety depersonalization syndrome. *Proceedings of the Royal Society of Medicine, 52,* 595–596.
4. Cattell, J. P., & Cattell, J. S. (1974). Depersonalization: psychological and social perspectives. In S. Arieti (Ed.), *American handbook of psychiatry* (pp. 767–799). Basic Books.
5. Harper, M., & Roth, M. (1962). Temporal lobe epilepsy and the phobic anxiety-depersonalization syndrome. *Comprehensive Psychiatry, 3,* 129–151.
6. Ambrosino, S. (1973). Phobic anxiety-depersonalization syndrome. *New York State Journal of Medicine, 73,* 419–425.
7. Simeon, D., Knutelska, M., Nelson, D., & Guralnik, O. (2003). Feeling unreal: A depersonalization disorder update of 117 cases. *Journal of Clinical Psychiatry, 64,* 990–997.
8. Hollander, E., Liebowitz, M. R., DeCaria, C., Fairbanks, J., Fallon, B., & Klein, D. F. (1990). Treatment of depersonalization with serotonin reuptake blockers. *Journal of Clinical Psychopharmacology, 10*(3), 200–203.
9. Ratliff, N. B., & Kerski, D. (1995). Depersonalization treated with fluoxetine. *American Journal of Psychiatry, 152*(11), 1689–1690.
10. Fichtner, C. G., Horevitz, R. P., & Braun, B. G. (1992). Fluoxetine in depersonalization disorder. *American Journal of Psychiatry, 149*(12), 1750–1751.
11. Simeon, D., Guralnik, O., Schmeidler, J., & Knutelska, M. (2004). Fluoxetine therapy in depersonalisation disorder: Randomised controlled trial. *British Journal of Psychiatry, 185,* 31–36.

12. Simeon, D., Stein, D. J., & Hollander, E. (1998). Treatment of depersonalization disorder with clomipramine. *Biological Psychiatry, 44*, 302–303.

13. Anand, A., Charney, D., Oren, D., Berman, R. M., Hu, X. S., Cappiello, A., & Krystal, J. H. (2000). Attenuation of the neuropsychiatric effects of ketamine with lamotrigine: Support for hyperglutamatergic effects of N-methyl-D-aspartate receptor antagonists. *Archives of General Psychiatry, 57*(3), 270–276.

14. Sierra, M., Phillips, M. L., Lambert, M. V., Senior, C., David, A. S., & Krystal, J. H. (2001). Lamotrigine in the treatment of depersonalization disorder. *Journal of Clinical Psychiatry, 62*(10), 826–827.

15. Sierra, M., Phillips, M. L., Krystal, J., & David, A. S. (2003). A placebo-controlled, crossover trial of lamotrigine in depersonalization disorder. *Journal of Psychopharmacology, 17*(1), 103–105.

16. Sierra, M., Baker, D., Medford, N., Lawrence, E., Patel, M., Phillips, M. L., & David, A. S. (2006). Lamotrigine as an add-on treatment for depersonalization disorder: A retrospective study of 32 cases. *Clinical Neuropharmacology, 29*(5), 253–258.

17. Aliyev, N. A., & Aliyev, Z. N. (2011). Lamotrigine in the immediate treatment of outpatients with depersonalization disorder without psychiatric comorbidity: Randomized, double-blind, placebo-controlled study. *Journal of Clinical Psychopharmacology, 31*(1), 61–65. [Retraction in: Shader, R. I., & Greenblatt, D. J. (2014). *Journal of Clinical Psychopharmacology, 34*(6), 671.]

18. Bohus, M. J., Landwehrmeyer, B., Stiglmayr, C. E., Limberger, M. F., Bohme, R., & Schmahl, C. G. (1999). Naltrexone in the treatment of dissociative symptoms in patients with borderline personality disorder: An open-label trial. *Journal of Clinical Psychiatry, 60*(9), 598–603.

19. Glover, H. (1993). A preliminary trial of nalmefene for the treatment of emotional numbing in combat veterans with post-traumatic stress disorder. *Israeli Journal of Psychiatry and Related Sciences, 30*(4), 255–263.

20. Nuller, Y. L., Morozova, M. G., Kushnir, O. N., & Hamper, N. (2001). Effect of naloxone therapy on depersonalization: A pilot study. *Journal of Psychopharmacology, 15*(2), 93–95.

21. Simeon, D., & Knutelska, M. (2005). An open trial of naltrexone in the treatment of depersonalization disorder. *Journal of Clinical Psychopharmacology, 25*, 267–270.

22. Pape, W., & Wöller, W. (2015). Low dose naltrexone in the treatment of dissociative symptoms. *Der Nervenarzt, 86*(3), 346–351. doi:10.1007/s00115-014-4015-9. PMID: 25421416

23. Gainer, D. M., Crawford, T. N., Fischer, K. B., & Wright, M. D. (2021). The relationship between dissociative symptoms and the medications used in the treatment of opioid use disorder. *Journal of Substance Abuse Treatment, 121*(February), 108195. doi: 10.1016/j.jsat.2020.108195

24. Mantovani, A., Simeon, D., Urban, N., Bulow, P., Allart, A., & Lisanby, S. (2011). Temporo-parietal junction stimulation in the treatment of depersonalization disorder. *Psychiatry Research, 186*, 138–140.

25. Christopeit, M., Simeon, D., Urban, N., Gowatsky, J., Lisanby, S. H., & Mantovani, A. (2014). Effects of repetitive transcranial magnetic stimulation (rTMS) on specific symptom clusters in depersonalization disorder. *Brain Stimulation, 7*(1), 141–143.

26. Jay, E.-L., Sierra, M., Van den Eynde, F., Rothwell, J. C., & David, A. S. (2014). Testing a neurobiological model of depersonalization disorder using repetitive transcranial magnetic stimulation. *Brain Stimulation, 7*, 252–259.

27. Jay, E.-L., Nestler, S., Sierra, M., McClelland, J., Kekic, M., & David, A..S. (2016). Ventrolateral prefrontal cortex repetitive transcranial magnetic stimulation in the treatment of depersonalization disorder: A consecutive case series. *Psychiatry Research, 240*, 118–122.

Chapter 12

1. Hunter, E. C. M., Phillips, M. L., Chalder, T., Sierra, M., & David, A. S. (2003). Depersonalisation disorder: A cognitive-behavioural conceptualization. *Behaviour Research and Therapy, 41*, 1451–1467.
2. Hunter, E. C. M., Baker, D., Phillips, M. L., Sierra, M., & David, A. S. (2005). Cognitive-behavioural therapy for depersonalisation disorder: An open study. *Behaviour Research and Therapy, 43*, 1121–1130.
3. Donnelly, K., & Neziroglu, F. (2010). *Overcoming depersonalization disorder: A mindfulness and acceptance guide to conquering feelings of numbness and unreality*. New Harbinger Publications, Inc.

Chapter 13

1. Bergler, E., & Eidelberg, L. (1938). The mechanism of depersonalization. *Psychoanalytic Review, 25*, 551.
2. Schilder, P. (1939). The treatment of depersonalization. *Bulletin of the New York Academy of Medicine, 15*, 258–272.
3. Cattell, J. P., & Cattell, J. S. (1974). Depersonalization: Psychological and social perspectives. In S. Arieti (Ed.), *American Handbook of Psychiatry* (pp 767–799). Basic Books.
4. Fewtrell, W. D. (1986). Depersonalisation: A description and suggested strategies. *British Journal of Guidance and Counselling, 14*, 263–269.
5. Levy, J. S., & Wachtel, P. L. (1978). Depersonalization: An effort at clarification. *American Journal of Psychoanalysis, 38*, 291–300.
6. Frances, A., Sacks, M., & Aronoff, M. S. (1977). Depersonalization: A self-relations perspective. *International Journal of Psychoanalysis, 58*(3), 325–331.
7. Fonagy, P., Gergely, G., Jurist, E. L., & Targe, M. (2004). *Affect regulation, mentalization, and the development of the self*. Other Press.
8. Putnam, F. W. (2016). *The way we are: How states of mind influence our identities, personality and potential for change*. Ipbooks
9. Horney, K. (1950). Neurosis and human growth, chapter 6, Alienation from self. In *Collected works of Karen Horney* (Vol. II, pp. 155–175). Norton.
10. Winnicott, D. W. (1960). Ego distortion in terms of true and false self. In D. W. Winnicott (Ed.), *The maturational processes and the facilitating environment: Studies in the theory of emotional development* (pp. 140–152). Karnac Books.
11. Kohut, H. (1973). *The restoration of the self*. International Universities Press, Inc.
12. Winnicott, D. W. (1965). *The maturational processes and the facilitating environment: Studies in the theory of emotional development*. Hogarth Press and Institute of Psycho-Analysis.
13. Ainsworth, M. D. S., & Bowlby, J. (1991). An ethological approach to personality development. *American Psychologist, 46*, 331–341.

14. Benjamin, J. (1990). An outline of intersubjectivity: The development of recognition. *Psychoanalytic Psychology, 7*(Suppl), 33–46.
15. Schilder, P. (1953). Ego and personality. In *Medical Psychology* (pp. 298–339). New York: International Universities Press.
16. Ambrosino, S. (1976). Depersonalization: A review and rethinking of a nuclear problem. *American Journal of Psychoanalysis, 36*(2), 105–118.
17. Winnicott, D. W. (1989). Basis for self in body. In C. Winnicott, R. Shepherd, & M. Davis (Eds.), *Psychoanalytic Explorations* (pp. 262–270). Cambridge, MA: Harvard University Press.
18. Fosha, D. (2013). A heaven in a wild flower: Self, dissociation, and treatment in the context of the neurobiological core self. *Psychoanalytic Inquiry, 33,* 496–523.
19. Michal, M., Adler, J., Wiltink, J., Reiner, I., Tschan, R., Wolfling, K., Weimert, S., Tuiin, I., Subic-Wrana, C., Beutel, M. E., & Zwerenz, R. (2016). A case series of 223 patients with depersonalization-derealization syndrome. *BMC Psychiatry, 16,* 203–213.
20. Simeon, D., Guralnik, O., Schmeidler, J., Sirof, B., & Knutelska, M. (2001). The role of childhood interpersonal trauma in depersonalization disorder. *American Journal of Psychiatry, 158,* 1027–1033.
21. Simeon, D., & Knutelska, M. (2022). The role of fearful attachment in depersonalization disorder. *European Journal of Trauma & Dissociation, 6,* 100266.
22. Wallin, D. J. (2007). *Attachment in psychotherapy.* Guilford Press.
23. McCullough, L., Kuhn, N., Andrews, S., Kaplan, A., Wolf, J., & Hurley, C. L. (2003). *Treating affect phobia: A manual for short-term dynamic psychotherapy.* Guilford Press.
24. Erikson, E. (1950). *Childhood and society.* Norton.
25. Havighurst, R. J. (1948). *Developmental tasks and education.* McKay.
26. Seiffge-Krenke, I., & Gelhaar, T. (2007). Does successful attainment of developmental tasks lead to happiness and success in later developmental tasks? A test of Havighurst's (1948) theses. *Journal of Adolescence, 31,* 33–52.
27. Guralnik, O., & Simeon, D. (2010). Depersonalization: Standing in the spaces between recognition and interpellation. *Psychoanalytic Dialogues, 20*(4), 400–416.
28. Chefetz, R. A. (2010). "T" in interpellation stands for terror: Commentary on paper by Orna Guralnik and Daphne Simeon. *Psychoanalytic Dialogues, 20*(4), 417–427.
29. LaMothe, R (2007). Beyond intersubjectivity: Personalization and community. *Psychoanalytic Psychology, 24*(2), 271–288.

Chapter 14

1. Turkle, S. (2011/2017). *Alone together: Why we expect more from technology and less from each other.* Basic Books.
2. Wallace, K. (2021, May 18). You are a network. *Aeon.* https://aeon.co/essays/the-self-is-not-singular-but-a-fluid-network-of-identities
3. Carr, N. (2010/2020). *The shallows: What the internet is doing to our brains.* W.W. Norton & Co. Inc.
4. Sklar, J. (2020, April 24). Zoom fatigue is taxing the brain. Here's why that happens. *National Geographic.* https://www.nationalgeographic.com/science/article/coronavirus-zoom-fatigue-is-taxing-the-brain-here-is-why-that-happens

5. Bezzubova, E. (2017). Virtual reality as a mirror of depersonalization. *Psychology Today*. https://www.psychologytoday.com/us/blog/the-search-self/201704/virtual-reality-mirror-depersonalization

6. Bezzubova, E. (2020). Virtual self and digital depersonalization: Between existential *Desein* and digital design. *Mind & Matter, 18*(1), 91–110.

7. Peckmann, C., Kannen, K., Pensel, M. C., Lux, S., Philipsen, A., & Braun, N. (2022). Virtual reality induces symptoms of depersonalization and derealization: A longitudinal randomized control trial. *Computers in Human Behavior, 131,* 107233.

8. Aardema, F., O'Connor, K., Côté, S., & Taillon, A. (2010). Virtual reality induces dissociation and lowers sense of presence in objective reality. *Cyberpsychology, Behavior, and Social Networking, 13*(4), 429–435.

9. Beech, M. (2020, March). COVID-19 pushes up internet use 70% and streaming more than 12%, first figures reveal. *Forbes*, https://www.forbes.com/sites/markbeech/2020/03/25/covid-19-pushes-up-internet-use-70-streaming-more-than-12-first-figures-reveal/?sh=312036f3104e.

10. Galanis, P., Vraka, I., Fragkou, D., Bilali, A., & Kaitelidou, D. (2021). Nurses' burnout and associated risk factors during the COVID-19 pandemic: A systematic review and meta-analysis. *Journal of Advanced Nursing, 77*(8), 3286–3302.

11. Miguel-Puga, J. A., Cooper-Bribiesca, D., Avelar-Garnica, F. J., Sanchez-Hurtado, L. A., Colin-Martínez, T., Espinosa-Poblano, E., Anda-Garay, J. C., González-Díaz, J. I., Segura-Santos, O. B., Vital-Arriaga, L. C., & Jáuregui-Renaud, K. (2021). Burnout, depersonalization, and anxiety contribute to post-traumatic stress in frontline health workers at COVID-19 patient care, a follow-up study. *Brain and Behavior, 11*(3), e02007.

12. Elhadi, M., Msherghi, A., Elgzairi, M., Alhashimi, A., Bouhuwaish, A., Biala, M., Abuelmeda, S., Khel, S., Khaled, A., Alsoufi, A., Elmabrouk, A., Bin Alshiteewi, F., Ben Hamed, T., Alhadi, B., Alhaddad, S., Elhadi, A., & Zaid, A. (2020). Burnout syndrome among hospital healthcare workers during the COVID-19 pandemic and civil war: A cross-sectional study. *Frontiers in Psychiatry, 11,* 579563.

13. Bezzubova, E. (2020). Digital depersonalization in the time of social isolation. *Psychology Today*. https://www.psychologytoday.com/us/blog/the-search-self/202005/digital-depersonalization-in-the-time-social-isolation

14. Ciaunica, A., McEllin, L., Kiverstein, J., Gallese, V., Hohwy, J., & Wozniak, M. (2022). Zoomed out? Depersonalization is related to increased digital media use during the COVID-19 pandemic lockdown. *Scientific Reports, 12*(3888), 15.

15. Schimmenti, A., Musetti, A., Costanzo, A., Terrone, G., Maganuco, N. R., Rinells, C. A., & Gervasi, A. M. (2019). The unfabulous four: Maladaptive personality functioning, insecure attachment, dissociative experiences and problematic internet use among young adults. *International Journal of Mental Health and Addiction, 19*, 447–461.

16. Maganuco, N. R., Constanzo, A., Midolo, L. R., Santoro, G., & Schimmenti, A. (2019). Impulsivity and alexithymia in virtual worlds: A study on players of World of Warcraft. *Clinical Neuropsychiatry: Journal of Treatment Evaluation, 16*(3), 127–134.

17. Muñoz, M. J., Fernández, L., & Gámez-Guadix, M. (2010). Analysis of the indicators of pathological Internet use in Spanish university students. *Spanish Journal of Psychology, 13*(2), 697–707.

18. Bernardi, S., & Pallanti, S. (2009). Internet addiction: A descriptive clinical study focusing on comorbidities and dissociative symptoms. *Comprehensive Psychiatry, 50*(6), 510–516.

19. Schimmenti, A., & Caretti, V. (2017). Video-terminal dissociative trance: Toward a psychodynamic understanding of problematic internet use. *Clinical Neuropsychiatry, 14,* 64–72.
20. Teo, A. R., & Gaw, A. C. (2010). Hikikomori, a Japanese culture-bound syndrome of social withdrawal? A proposal for DSM-5. *Journal of Nervous and Mental Disease, 198*(6), 444–449.

Index

For the benefit of digital users, indexed terms that span two pages (e.g., 52–53) may, on occasion, appear on only one of those pages.

Figures are indicated by *f* following the page number